T0184256

Community Health Care's *O*-Process for Evaluation

Community Health Care's *O*-Process for Evaluation

A Participatory Approach for Increasing Sustainability

Fannie Fonseca-Becker, DrPH, MPH
Johns Hopkins University

Amy L. Boore, PhD, MPH
Johns Hopkins University

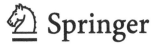 Springer

Fannie Fonseca-Becker
Johns Hopkins University
Bloomberg School of Public Health
Department of Health, Behavior and Society
111 Market Place, Suite 310
Baltimore, MD 21202

Amy L. Boore
Johns Hopkins University
Bloomberg School of Public Health
Department of Health, Behavior and Society
111 Market Place, Suite 310
Baltimore, MD 21202

ISBN: 978-0-387-77376-6   e-ISBN: 978-0-387-77377-3
DOI: 10.1007/978-0-387-77377-3

Library of Congress Control Number: 2008921356

Printed on acid-free paper

9 8 7 6 5 4 3 2 1

springer.com

Foreword

There is a renewed sense of urgency to alleviate human suffering and public attention has increased its focus on corporate philanthropy and social investing. Likewise, non-profit organizations find themselves under greater pressure to demonstrate impact and the demand for greater 'transparency' on the donor community and government agencies now require a more transparent accounting of spending on social programs that support the disenfranchised. This book is intended to be a guide for Community Health Care Programs interested in enhancing their long-term sustainability through the appropriate use of their evaluation results. The book has been designed for ease of use and provides step-by-step guidance on all aspects of basic evaluation methods.

For the last twenty years, The Johnson & Johnson Community Health Care Program has awarded funding to more than 150 pioneering non-profit organizations for unique projects that address disparities in America's delivery of health care to poor and underserved citizens. By supporting essential, community-based health care organizations, the program helps to break down health care barriers for medically underserved populations by improving their access to quality services. Assessing the effectiveness of the grantees efforts in increasing access to quality care is a cornerstone of the J&J Community Health Care Program. However, community-based organizations may require some assistance to collect, organize, and present in an optimally useful manner the information needed to provide to multiple audiences evidence of effectiveness in providing quality care. To fill this gap, the Johns Hopkins University Bloomberg School of Public Health has, since 1998, collaborated with Johnson & Johnson to provide the J&J Grantees with technical assistance in evaluation.

The partnership between the Johns Hopkins University Bloomberg School of Public Health and Johnson & Johnson was created to leverage an important academic-industry partnership in order to contribute to the long term sustainability of community health care programs by helping them increase their in-house capacity in monitoring and evaluation.

We encourage community health care organizations around the country to consider this book as a road map toward increasing their long-term-sustainability by measuring the effect of their programs and tailoring presentation of results to different audiences.

David Holtgrave, PhD
Professor and Chair,
Department of Health, Behavior and Society
Bloomberg School of Public Health
Johns Hopkins University

Rick A. Martinez, MD
Medical Director,
Corporate Contributions and
    Community Relations
Director,
Latin American Contributions
Johnson & Johnson

Acknowledgements

The "Community Health Care's 'O-Process for Evaluation'™: A Participatory Approach for Increasing Sustainability" was produced as a result of experience gained over the years since the inception of the J&J Community Health Care Scholars Program (J&J Scholars Program) at the Johns Hopkins University, Bloomberg School of Public Health. Dr. Fonseca-Becker, an Associate Scientist in the Department of Health, Behavior and Society and Director of the J&J Scholars Program, has trained and supervised over 40 doctoral students and their community health care projects in participatory evaluation methodologies. Dr. Amy Boore is with the Epidemiology Information Service at the Centers for Disease Control and Prevention in Atlanta and was, during the writing of this book, a doctoral candidate in the Department of Epidemiology at the Johns Hopkins Bloomberg School of Public Health. She also was a J&J Community Health Care Scholar and provided technical assistance to a J&J community health care grantee in Alabama.

The J&J Scholars Program is part of a collaboration between the Johnson and Johnson Community HealthCare Program and the Johns Hopkins Bloomberg School of Public Health to provide technical assistance in monitoring and evaluation to the J&J Community Health Care Program grantees.

The authors thank Dr. Rick Martinez, Medical Director for Corporate Contributions and Community Relations, and Ms. Joanne Fillweber, Manager for Medical Affairs and Corporate Contributions at Johnson & Johnson for their continued support and unwavering dedication to improving and increasing access to quality health care for underserved populations around the country.

The authors also thank the dedicated J&J Scholars who field-tested earlier versions of this document including, Ling Shi, MD, Sarah Shea, MPH, Sarah Szanton, MSN, PhD, Thomas Guadamuz, MHS, PhD and Amy Vastine, MPH, PhD. We are indebted to Professor Stan Becker for his critique and comments, and to Dr. David Holtgrave for his encouragement and endorsement. We also thank, Ms. Mary Lemon, for her administrative support and attention to detail.

Contents

4   Organize & Analyze Data

5   Outputs & Outcomes

Appendix 1 Data Collection Tools

Appendix 2 Worksheets

Introduction

Fannie Fonseca-Becker and Amy L. Boore

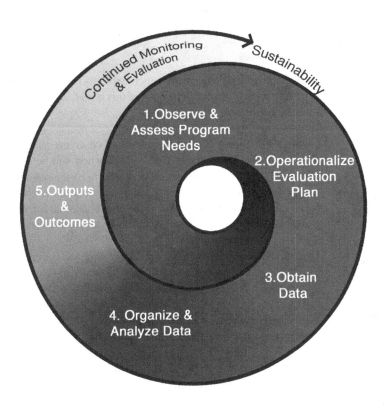

The "*O*-Process" for Evaluation

Evaluation does not have to be complex. If you would like to track the progress of your program, make sure it is being implemented as planned, or determine if it is meeting its objectives, you may want to conduct the evaluation on your own (rather than hire an external evaluator). The "*O*-process©" for evaluation was developed to serve as a simple reference to help lead you through the necessary steps to conduct your own in-house evaluation.

The "*O*-Process" contains five basic steps:

1. Observe & assess your program needs,
2. Operationalize and design the evaluation plan,
3. Obtain data,
4. Organize & analyze the data, and
5. Report Outputs and Outcomes.

Each step corresponds to a chapter in this book, which explains how to perform the step in detail. By following these steps with the help of this guide, any program can conduct its own in-house evaluation.

Chapter 1 will help outline the process of observing and assessing program needs. The different types of evaluation will be described, along with possible reasons for conducting each. By the end of module 1, you should have a clear idea of what your program hopes to gain from an evaluation, what type of evaluation is feasible for your program, and what type or types of evaluation you will conduct.

Chapter 2 leads you through operationalizing and designing your evaluation plan. It is important to think through all future steps of an evaluation and put them into a written plan. This will help the full evaluation process go according to plan and produce the results you need. By the end of Chapter 2, you should have a well-defined plan for the remaining parts of the evaluation.

Chapter 3 covers how to obtain data for your evaluation. Different types of evaluation or different levels of resources available will determine what types of information are important to collect. Tools for collecting the information are also provided. By the end of Chapter 3 you should be able to find and gather the data you need for your evaluation.

Chapter 4 describes how to organize and analyze the data you have collected. There are many ways to describe the data you collect, ranging from very simple to very complex. This Chapter will provide tools for doing basic analysis of your data. By the end of Chapter 4, you should be able to describe your data using simple statistics, graphs, and charts.

Chapter 5 leads you through the decisions you need to make regarding what to do with your results – the outputs and outcomes of your evaluation. It is important the results from all the work you do in the evaluation get used for some good, either by your own project or by others. By the end of Chapter 5, you should have a clear idea of how to report your results, and who should see and use the results.

Conducting an evaluation is all about decisions. What type of evaluation to choose, when and where to conduct it, what information to collect, how to report the results, etc. For that reason, each Chapter in this guide will begin will a decision-making tree. These will allow you to follow through the decision making process for each step, and determine what parts of the guide you should refer to next.

Although the decision making trees are positioned at the beginning of each Chapter, it is not expected that you will be able or prepared to answer each of the questions posed in them right away. The rest of the Chapter is designed to help you figure out how to answer each step in the tree. By working through the Chapter, you will be able to move down through the decision making process and further clarify your evaluation plan.

Evaluation, like an "*O*," is a continual process. Each step leads into another, but it is a process that should not end with the last step. The results from evaluation can help you strengthen your program, but sustainability can only be achieved if you continue to improve and adapt the program through continued evaluation.

Some forms of evaluation, such as impact evaluation (which will be described in Chapter 1), require more sophisticated evaluation designs. Although they still follow the five steps of the "*O*-Process," they require more time, resources, and expertise in evaluation. For these, you will probably need to hire an external evaluator. It is still very important, however, to read through the steps of the "O-Process" and understand the basic elements of evaluation. This will help you guide the evaluator and ensure that you get the results you need.

Before you can begin on the "*O*-Process" or the rest of this guide, it is important to make sure you have a clear definition for your program, that you have identified stakeholders, and that you have some idea of the program's goals and objectives.

Chapter 1
Observe & Assess Program Needs

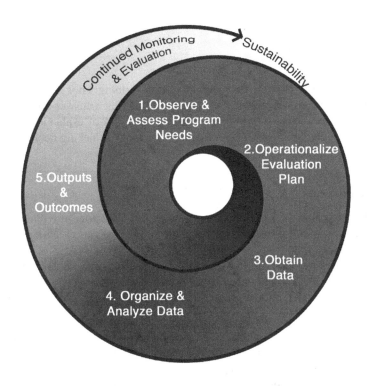

Contents

Observe & Assess Program Needs

This chapter will help you clarify how evaluation can fit into your programs. By the end of this chapter, you will be able to describe the main types of evaluation, determine which types are possible and desirable for your program, identify your program's stakeholders, and continue forward to build an evaluation plan.

> Evaluation is a way to show that your program is doing what it is supposed to be doing

What Is Evaluation?

Evaluation is a way to show that your program is doing what it is supposed to be doing. There are many types of evaluation, all of which answer different questions and require different levels of resources. All types of evaluation, however, involve the regular collection of information as a tool for making decisions about the program.

> **Evaluation can:**
> - Help you plan the best way to organize and conduct your program
> - Help you decide whether your resources are being used in the most efficient way
> - Show whether your program activities are being carried out as planned
> - Show whether or not your program is meeting its goals

Evaluation should not be considered an outside or extra option for your programs. Instead, evaluation should be considered an integral piece of the program, built into the program design right from the very beginning.

Program evaluation is like having a rearview mirror for your project. It allows you to see how things are going, identify potential threats, and adjust your course if need be. In other words, evaluation allows you to fully understand the effects of your program, so that you can better plan its future direction.

Why Do Evaluation?

Evaluation is not only beneficial to your program, it is quite often essential. Evaluation is necessary for several reasons:

To Show the Program Really Works

As an example of how important evaluation is, consider the following example. Southern Primary HealthCare Clinics, a nonprofit working to decrease cardiovascular disease (CVD) in the surrounding communities, conducts a two year health prevention program.

At the end of the two years, if the project had not conduct an evaluation of their efforts, are able to report the following:

> During the 2 years of our program, we enrolled 60 clients into the CVD prevention program. At the end of the program, many of the participants stated that they had lost weight and reduced their blood pressure. All of the participants enjoyed the program and stated that they would like it to continue

The question that should immediately spring to mind is, "but did it work?" Despite the professed reduction in blood pressure of "many participants," how much did their blood pressure actually improve? How much weight did participants generally lose? Were those that enrolled already at high risk to begin with? While the above anecdotal information is valuable, without having conducted an evaluation this project is unable to give a complete story of how and if the program really worked.

Now, consider if Southern Primary HealthCare Clinics had conducted an evaluation of their program. This time, at the end of two years they are able to report the following:

> During the 2 years of our program, we enrolled 60 clients into the CVD prevention program. All 60 were diagnosed as hypertensive before enrollment, and were referred by their primary physician as being at high risk for CVD. After the first year, 15 participants (25%) had reduced their blood pressure by 13 points. By the end of the second year, 25 participants (41.7%) had reduced their blood pressure by at least 13 points, and 18 (30%) had achieved normal blood pressure (systolic <120 mmHg and diastolic <80 mmHg). Of the 18 achieving normal blood pressure, 12 had reported at baseline that they had unsuccessfully tried to reduce their blood pressure on their own in the past. All participants stated that they enjoyed the program and would like it to continue.

By conducting an evaluation, the program was able to give a much more complete story of how the program worked. It is also possible for the project staff to determine whether the results were as expected, or whether the program is doing better or worse than originally planned.

Any program that hopes to succeed in the long term must be open to the idea of improvement. Even a highly successful program may end up with diminishing returns over time if it fails to keep up with social trends, shifts in the target population, or other changes in the community.

Regardless of whether your program is targeting CVD or any other community health problem, it is critical that you have some measure of whether the program is working according to plan. Think about the following questions:

- Is the message you are sending to the target population being heard and interpreted as you had hoped?
- Is the population most in need of your intervention the one most likely to obtain it?
- Is your program achieving its goals?
- Are there unexpected barriers or unexpected results?
- In short—can you *show* that the program works?

If your program has ever had the need to answer any of those questions evaluation, can help you find the most complete and compelling answers.

To Strengthen the Program

Sometimes, evaluation reveals that the program is falling short of its goals. Since evaluation involves keeping careful records, it is possible to then go back and identify weak spots in the program.

Answering "yes" or "no" to the questions at the top of this page show you whether the program works. Knowing *why* the answers are either "yes" or "no" will help you strengthen the program. Evaluation can give you the reasons why.

To Satisfy Donor Requirements

Many donor agencies add program evaluation as a requirement of the funding grant. While some do not specify the type of evaluation that must be done, others require a particular type of evaluation. Making evaluation a consistent and integral part of your programs from the beginning will make it easier to satisfy these requirements, and will give you more complete (and convincing) results to report to donors.

To Gain Additional Funding

In addition to satisfying the requirements of donors who have already agreed to fund your programs, program evaluation can help you obtain new funding. A grant application that spells out an organized evaluation plan is far more competitive than one that makes little mention of evaluation. A well-thought-out evaluation plan shows that a program is looking ahead and is open to improvement. Donors also want to know their funds are well spent and, without an evaluation plan to provide them with this information, they may be wary to invest the funds.

To Influence Policy

Community health programs work to fulfill unmet needs in the populations they serve. It is important to show policy makers that the needs exist and that the program is having a beneficial effect on the community. Influencing positive policy decisions can sometimes be the most substantial and long-lasting contribution a program can make. Policy makers can be hard to convince, however. Without conducting an evaluation of the program, it is much more difficult to get the numbers and figures that policy makers rely on when making decisions.

To Inform the Community & Other Organizations

It is also important to show the community, your own project staff and board of directors, and other organizations what worked or didn't work about your program. Community leaders are likely to appreciate getting information on how your program is working, and may have suggestions if parts of the program are not meeting their goals. Having and reporting the information collected from evaluation can help foster collaborations with other organizations and help you decide whether the program merits replication in other communities. Your overall goal is, after all, to improve health for communities. Knowing exactly what effect your program has on community health, and sharing that information with others, is a very powerful way to increase your positive impact on communities.

What Evaluation Can Do for Your Program

Different types of evaluation are able to help your program in different ways. In this book, we describe the most basic types of evaluation.

Formative evaluation asks:
  What is the best way to run the program?

Process evaluation asks:
  Is the program running the way we planned it to?

Outcome evaluation asks:
  Is the program meeting its goals? Is it making a difference?

Formative Evaluation

This type of evaluation is conducted before the program is started. **Formative evaluation guides the design and implementation of the program.** It tells you about the health related problems that your program will address, and the best way to implement your program to have the greatest impact on the health problems.

Process Evaluation

This type of evaluation should be started before the program is implemented and then carried on through the end of the program. **Process evaluation is used to determine how well the program is implemented**. It tells you whether the program is going as planned, and helps identify unexpected barriers or problems. Process evaluation is used to fine-tune your program to make it more efficient and to help it have the greatest impact.

Outcome Evaluation

This type of evaluation is performed after the program has been operating long enough that it could be reasonably expected to have created some changes in the community. **Outcome evaluation is used to determine if your program is meeting its goals and objectives.** There are two main types of outcome evaluation; *intermediate* and *impact*. Intermediate outcome evaluation tells you whether the program has met its objectives. Impact evaluation shows whether the changes seen in the community can actually be attributed to the program.

> For intermediate outcome evaluation, it is possible (though not preferable) to conduct the evaluation even if no information had previously been collected on the program.
>
> For impact evaluation, however, you *must* have collected baseline information before (or at the time of) program initiation.

Impact evaluation will help you to show that your project—and not any other circumstances or trends in the community—were responsible for the positive changes in your target population. As this type of evaluation demands some fairly sophisticated study designs, however, it is beyond the scope of this book to describe in detail.

The following simple diagram shows the usual timing of each main type of evaluation during the life of a program.

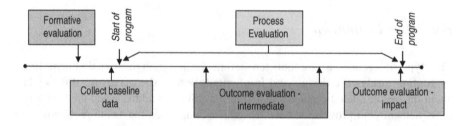

> Resources on impact evaluation and on hiring external evaluators to help you with an impact evaluation are listed in the references section at the end of the book.

Unlike formative or process evaluation, it is important that an outcome evaluation not be conducted too early. Since the goal of any outcome evaluation is to determine whether the program is meeting its goals and making a difference, you must be careful to allow enough time for the program to actually accomplish these things. Otherwise, the evaluation will likely show that your program is not meeting its objectives, when the truth may be that it just hasn't had enough time to do so yet.

Other Types of Evaluation

Other kinds of evaluation that you may have heard of or want to use include *cost-benefit analysis, cost-effectiveness analysis,* and *social network analysis.* These generally require an external evaluator, so they are not covered in this book.

> The reference list includes some other resources with information about different types of evaluation, such as social network or costbenefit analysis.

Assessing Which Type of Evaluation Meets Your Needs

What type of evaluation is best for your program depends on several factors, including:

- The stage of development of the program;
- What information you already collect on program activities (if the program has already started);
- The financial and staff resources available;
- The needs and desires of stakeholders (including your own program staff).

The following decision-making tree may be useful to help decide which types of evaluation would be good for your program (Fig. 1.1). The level of resources needed varies greatly depending on which type of evaluation you choose and what activities you plan to do as part of the evaluation. In general, process evaluation requires the least amount of resources and should be feasible for almost any small organization. Formative and outcome evaluations require more resources, especially in terms of staff time.

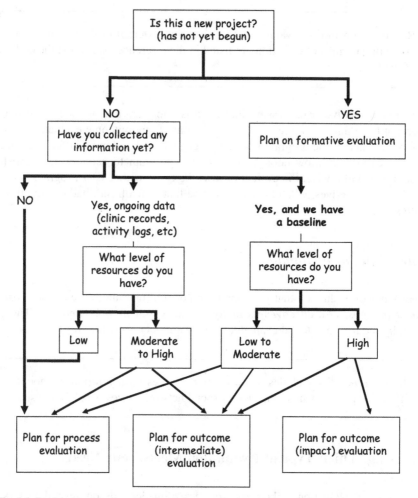

Fig. 1.1 Decision-making tree for choosing an evaluation type

A "baseline" refers to information collected before your program starts. It's a "starting point," that shows the situation before your program begins its work. Comparing it to information gathered later can show many changes have occurred since your program started.

In general, consider your project

A "Low" resource project if:
• You have less than five staff members or
• The amount you are able to devote to evaluation is less than 5% of the annual project budget

A "Moderate" resource project if:
- You have less than ten staff members or
- The amount you are able to devote to evaluation is less than 10% of the annual project budget

A "High" resource project if:
- You have greater staff and financial resources than mentioned above.

For a "full" evaluation, which includes all of the components outlined above (formative, process, intermediate outcome and impact), the general rule of thumb is that an amount equal to around 10% of the annual project budget should be set aside for the evaluation.

> It is usually best to commit to the more basic types of evaluation (formative if the program is has not started, process for either a new or ongoing program), and then decide whether to add the more complicated outcome evaluation designs based on available resources and stakeholder needs.

Just because you are unable to do a full evaluation, however, does **not** mean that you shouldn't do any evaluation at all. It is very common for projects to decide they want to do an evaluation for a program that has already begun and that has a limited budget. In this case, both process and intermediate outcome evaluations are possible.

This book details what is basically an "abbreviated" form of evaluation. It is perfectly acceptable to perform this type of simplified evaluation to help strengthen the programs you already have in place. It is highly recommended, however, that you write in the cost of doing full evaluations for programs you begin in the future.

Users of Evaluation Results

When deciding on an evaluation plan, it is important to consider who will use the results and how. People who are interested in your results and that may have some use for the results are your *stakeholders*.

It is extremely important to identify and involve your stakeholders from the beginning of the evaluation plans. Otherwise, you may hit unnecessary roadblocks in the implementation of your evaluation, or your stakeholders may not accept or believe your results.

So who are your stakeholders and what might they want to know from an evaluation? Consider the following list of possible stakeholders. Which ones are relevant to your program?

- ❑ Program staff & managers
- ❑ Program Board of Directors
- ❑ Program participants
- ❑ Volunteers
- ❑ Funders/Donors
- ❑ Community leaders
- ❑ Community organizations
- ❑ Parent groups
- ❑ Universities or high schools
- ❑ State or local health departments
- ❑ Hospitals or medical clinics
- ❑ Local healthcare providers
- ❑ Other nonprofit organizations in the area
- ❑ Other people working on similar issues
- ❑ Policy makers
- ❑ Local government / politicians
- ❑ Media
- ❑ Governmental agencies
- ❑ Local or national partners
- ❑ Special interest groups
- ❑ Religious organizations
- ❑ Private businesses or business groups
- ❑ Groups critical of the program
- ❑ Law enforcement agencies

Each stakeholder or group of stakeholders may have very different questions or desires for an evaluation. Also on the next page are some examples of what a few common stakeholders often want to learn from an evaluation.

Stakeholder: Funders/donors

Question	Evaluation type
• How will funds be allocated during the program?	Formative
• It the program designed in a way that it is most likely to achieve its objectives?	
• Are funds being used efficiently?	Process
• Have program activities been carried out as planned?	
• Did the program work?	Outcome
• Should the program continue to be funded, or be replicated or expanded?	

Stakeholder: Community leaders

Question	Evaluation type
• What is the goal of the program?	Formative
• Does the program address an issue that the community considers a priority?	
• What exactly the program is doing (what services are provided, who is involved, how to access the services, etc).	Process
• Does the program work?	Outcome

Stakeholder: Program staff

Question	Evaluation type
• What is needed for program implementation?	Formative
• Is the program truly wanted or needed in the community?	
• What are the strengths and weaknesses of the program?	Process
• Are there unanticipated barriers that may be preventing the program from carrying out its activities as planned?	
• Does the program really make a difference?	Outcome

In addition to these very broad examples, your stakeholders will very likely have questions specific to your program or your community. The only way to know what your stakeholders want from an evaluation is to ask them.

Once you begin planning an evaluation, send a brief letter to your stakeholders and inform them about the upcoming evaluation. Make it clear that you are soliciting their support and their input, and give an easy way for them to send feedback.

> Make sure to send a "thank you" to stakeholders who respond to you with feedback. Let them know that you value their input and will take it into serious consideration, but that you may not be able to incorporate all feedback into your evaluation.

You will not be able to satisfy the desires of all of your stakeholders, and should also make that clear in any communication you send them. But hearing all of their feedback and concerns can give you a good direction and some good ideas for your evaluation. Chapter 2 of this book provides more detail about involving stakeholders in the design and conduct of your evaluation.

Roadblocks to Evaluation

Despite the importance of evaluation to community health programs, they are often not conducted. While it is true that evaluation is not a simple task, barriers that are often perceived by organizations as being insurmountable can usually be overcome relatively easily. A few of the more common roadblocks, along with suggested solutions, are listed below.

"We don't have the Resources for Evaluation"

Different kinds of evaluation require different amounts of resources. The most basic forms of evaluation require very little extra time or budget. In fact, you are probably already conducting process evaluation activities without even knowing it. Does your project keep track of the number of clients served, seminars given, community meetings attended, pamphlets distributed, doctors visits scheduled, etc? These are inexpensive and easy tasks to perform, and they are absolutely essential for a program to stay organized and accountable.

Lack of resources may require you to stick with basic process evaluation at first. **It is best to only do what your resources allow, as otherwise you may not be able to complete the evaluation or may not be able to get good data, which could cause frustration and impede future evaluation efforts**. When you submit

grants for extra funding for the program or start a new program, incorporate extra
amounts for a more in-depth evaluation.

"Evaluation is Too Judgmental. We don't want our Program to be Judged as a 'Bad' Program"

Many community organizations avoid evaluation because they are worried about
the consequences of "negative" results. While it is possible that an evaluation will
show weaknesses in the program, this should not be cause for alarm. It is just as
important (or actually more so) to discover the program weaknesses as it is to discover its strengths. **You want to make sure your program is being as effective as
possible. Evaluation can help you to figure out what is not working quite right,
and can guide you in making improvements.** Rather than fear any changes that
evaluation might bring about, resolve to use evaluation results—whether "positive"
or "negative"—as agents for change in a *positive direction.*

In-house evaluation Vs. External evaluators

Benefits of in-house evaluation:

- Increases capacity of staff for future evaluations
- Staff know the program the best, have better understanding of what
  evaluation needs to show
- Requires less financial resources Benefits of external evaluators:
- Benefits of external evalucations:
- Able to conduct more sophisticated types of evaluation
- More objective, "outsider's" perspective on program
- Requires less time from program staff

"We Would Need to Hire an Outside Evaluator Since we've Never Done an Evaluation Before"

While it is true that evaluation often requires people with certain skills sets, **it is
quite possible for small community-based organizations to conduct their own
in-house evaluation.** This guide is meant to be a first step toward conducting simple forms of evaluation. If your program has the funds to hire an outside evaluator,
that is an option to consider. Outside evaluators can help you to conduct more
in-depth forms of evaluation. Even if you do hire an outside evaluator, you should
have an understanding of how evaluation works. Only then can you help guide the
evaluator and make sure that the evaluation suits the needs of your program and
your stakeholders.

The key to conducting an in-house evaluation without an expert evaluator on the staff is to make the evaluation a collaborative effort. Through discussion and sharing of ideas, the different members of your team can combine their own unique talents and build their skills through learning from each other.

"It Takes too much Staff Time for an Evaluation"

Gaining staff support for evaluation can be one of the more challenging roadblocks to evaluation. Not wanting extra work, feeling as if there's no time, or feeling that it is already "known" that the project works and is thus unnecessary to conduct an evaluation are all common sentiments. And it's true that evaluation requires work, and takes time. It may also be true that you and your staff "know" the program works. But others (donors, community members, politicians, etc) may not take your word for it—they want *evidence* that the program works.

The key to gaining staff support is to *involve them*. The program staff is your most important groups of stakeholders, and staff members should be involved in the decision-making process along with other stakeholders. By giving staff and other stakeholders a say in the evaluation, they acquire a sense of ownership and commitment to the evaluation. Not only will this increase support, but it will also help to relieve fears about how evaluation results will be used.

Chapter 1 checklist—Observe & Assess Program Needs
_____
❑ Clear idea of what evaluation is and its value
❑ Decision made on type of evaluation to conduct and why
❑ Identification & involvement of stakeholders
❑ Acknowledgment of obstacles/roadblocks to evaluation

Chapter 2
Operationalize the Evaluation Plan

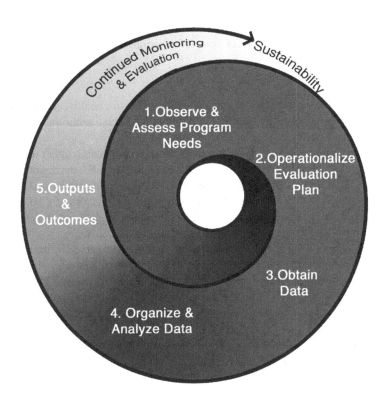

Contents

Operationalize the Evaluation Plan

This chapter will help you to operationalize your evaluation plan. That means putting together a plan for your evaluation that is clear and achievable, and that meets your program needs.

Building an evaluation plan requires a fair amount of brainstorming and coordination, setting deadlines, and assigning responsibilities to each member of your team. There are many other important components, and therefore this will be one of the longer chapters of this book.

Throughout this chapter and the remainder of the book, the Southern Primary HealthCare Clinic example will be used to illustrate certain points. Although this is a fictitious organization and program, the case study was built using examples from several existing organizations and government survey data. A general summary of the case study is provided below for your information.

Southern Primary HealthCare Clinics is a comprehensive health care provider serving approximately 3,000 patients in two clinics for three semirural counties in a Southeast Sate.

Cardiovascular disease is higher in the Southeast compared to other regions of the country. Health disparities in this State parallel those for the region with the African American population being at greater risk for disability and early death from CVD than the white population. Major risk factors of CVD that can be modified or treated include high blood pressure, high blood cholesterol levels, obesity, and overweight and physical inactivity.

The majority (70%) of the population in the three counties served by the clinics are African American. A large proportion (40%) of the population served lives at 200% of the poverty level, 35% are uninsured, and approximately 15% of the adults have less than a tenth- grade education. Almost half of the clinic's clients are at high risk for CVD, with 48% being obese, 42% having high blood cholesterol levels, and 39% of women and 37% of men having high blood pressure.

To address some of the risk factors associated with CVD, the Southern Primary HealthCare clinics received a 2-year grant to develop and implement a Cardiovascular Disease Prevention and Control (CVDPC) program. The goal of the CVDPC program is to prevent and control CVD among the adult population served by the Southern Primary HealthCare Clinics.

The CVDPC program is based on the Healthy People 2010 goals specific to the prevention of heart disease. In the CVDPC program the routine health care provided by the medical doctor treating the client is enhanced by health education sessions, enrollment in a subsidized drug program, peer support groups, home visitations, and walking groups.

Although your program is likely different than the Southern Primary HealthCare Clinics, use of this example will hopefully help to illustrate key points in this manual and allow you to think through the components of evaluation as they apply to your own program.

Select an Evaluation Team

Conducting an evaluation is a little like doing detective work. The evidence is there, and it's your job to figure out how to collect it, what to do with it, and how to put it all together to tell the story of what happened.

> If you were a detective, you would want your investigative team to have a wide range of specialties (such as forensic specialist, expert interrogator, media relations specialist, etc). It is the same for your evaluation team. You will need people who are good at different things, and who bring different ideas to the evaluation.

Your program will need an evaluation director, who will be in charge of coordinating all of the evaluation work. Since evaluation is too big a job for just one person, decide who else will be on the "evaluation team." Three or four people are usually sufficient to get started. Later you may need to temporarily recruit more people for some specific tasks that require more manpower or more expertise.

If you have a choice of people (not all projects do), try to get a good mix of staff. The key is to have people who can bring different perspectives and ideas to the table. You especially want:

- Someone who actually interacts with the clients (i.e., nurses, caseworkers, drivers, educators, etc.). Do you have that person that just seems to know *everyone*? You may want to choose that person for your evaluation team.
- Someone with good writing and organizational skills, to keep records and write the evaluation reports.
- Someone who has a good working knowledge of the people, material, and financial resources available at the program. This may be a higher-level project supervisor or it may just be that person who always seems to know everything about your project.

The following decision-making tree may also be useful in deciding on your evaluation team (Fig. 2.1).

In addition to staff members, consider inviting key community leaders, clients of your program, or others who could bring a different perspective on your program and its place in the community to the team. You might be surprised at how much a fresh perspective can help you conduct the evaluation, not to mention the increased support such representation would lend to your evaluation from the community or target population.

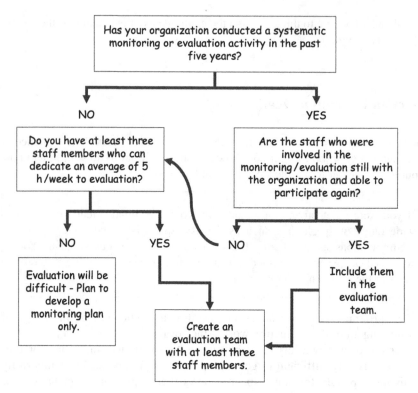

Fig. 2.1 Monitoring or evaluation decision tree

> Choose an interesting program or one that is likely easy to evaluate for your
> first evaluation. This will hold the interest of your team, and getting positive
> results can empower your organization and fuel interest in conducting further
> evaluations.

Many organizations have more than one program going on at the same time. Each
program will likely require a separate evaluation, so choose just one to focus on for
your first evaluation. Choose a program that is a highlight of your organization, or one
that has a lot of interest from the community or your staff. That way, the first evaluation will be an exciting one that is likely to give you positive results.

Review What Your Program Is Targeting

It is imperative that your evaluation team has a clear definition of the problem that
your program is to address. Phrase it in terms of the underlying **problem**, not the
need itself. An example of *need* would be "the community needs a substance

abuse program," or "the community lacks a substance abuse program." These two statements are not helpful in guiding your evaluation efforts. They state what your program may *provide,* but not what it *targets.*

When considering why it's better to state the problem than the need, think about how your results will sound to outside persons.

Which is more convincing:
"Through providing a substance abuse program, our program was able to meet the need in the community to have such a program"
or
"Through providing a substance abuse program, our program was able to help decrease substance abuse among our clients by 15%"

A better statement would describe the underlying *problem,* such as, "there is a high rate of substance abuse in the community." This last statement most clearly defines what the evaluation will be measuring, as it is the *problem* that your program is ultimately targeting. To show your program works, you will need to show that there has been an improvement in the problem.

Southern Primary HealthCare Example

What is the problem in the community that this program will address?
Many adults living in the communities served by our clinics are at high risk for CVD.

How did you become aware of this issue?
National statistics from the CDC show the rate of CVD as being higher in our area than in other regions of the USA. 30% of patients reporting to our clinics suffer from CVD, and half of our clients have been labeled by their physicians as being "at risk."

Who is directly affected?	How are they affected?
Those with CVD	Suffer poor health, earlier deaths
Families of those with CVD Communities	Emotional & financial burden, loss of loved ones Detracts from community life & economic well-being to have adults in poor health
Medical institutions	Increased burden of caring for patients with CVD
State	Economic loss due to health care costs & loss of otherwise productive adults
What are some possible reasons for this problem? Higher rates of blood cholesterol and hypertension in community members	**Why do these reasons exist?** Poor diets / obesity
	Decreased physical exercise
Increased rates of obesity in community	Lack of affordable healthy food choices
	Decreased physical exercise
Decreased physical exercise	Increased work hours among low-income families
	Increased TV watching/ indoor activities

Smoking	High stress among lower-income families
	Social norm for young adults
Diabetes	Overweight / obesity
	Genetic predisposition

How has this problem changed over the past several years? *(general trend in community)*	What influences have led to the changes? Diets/nutritional habits worsening
Increasing rates of CVD in the community	Crime increase=decrease in outdoor exercise
(who is affected)	Increase in obesity rates
Increasingly common in women	Higher rates of female smokers
(funding levels—public or private sources)	Cutbacks in government-subsidized programs
Government funding has dropped, private funding about the same	Private funding initiatives
(attention paid—media, schools, other)	Concerns over obesity rates in children
Attention is on obesity epidemic	CVD not mentioned much in media or other general information sources
(similar changes elsewhere in country?)	Diets/nutritional habits worsening
Similar elsewhere, and increasing especially in minority/low-income areas of the country	

Who else is working on this?	What have they done?	Has it been successful?
"Healthy hearts, healthy minds" program	Educational programs for adults with chronic disease or depression	Unknown
	Help register qualified patients for Medicaid	More people are enrolled in program than one year ago?

Define Program Goals and Objectives

A program *must* define its goals and objectives. Even if you have previously defined your goals & objectives, take some time to review them with your evaluation team to make sure everyone is on the same track. This is also a good step to engage your stakeholders, and you may be surprised to find out that not all stakeholders agree on what the goals or objectives of your program are!

Use the following decision-making tree to help you as you go through defining your goals and objectives (Fig. 2.2).

A Goal is:

A general statement of what the program is trying to accomplish.

- General expectation
- Can be vague
- May not be measurable

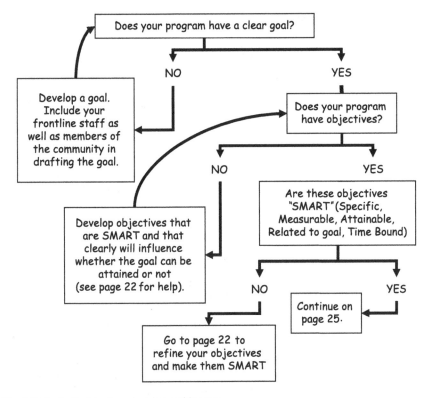

Fig. 2.2 Goals & objectives decision making tree

An objective is:

A specific statement of expected results

- Always measurable
- The means by which the goals are met

A program goal is basically its mission or purpose. A goal is a statement of what you hope to achieve through the program. It is usually very broad, and may not be directly measurable.

The goal of Southern Primary HealthCare Clinic's Cardiovascular Disease Prevention and Control Program is to prevent and control CVD among the adult population served by the project's two clinics.

An *objective* is a statement of expected or intended change over a given time frame. If you are doing a process evaluation, your objectives will focus on changes in program activities and utilization of your program services. If you are performing an outcome evaluation, the objectives will focus on changes in the health status of the target population.

Southern Primary HealthCare Clinics CVDPC **process** objectives:

- Increase by 60% the number of eligible hypertensive clients who participate in the CVDPC Program by the end of year 2.
- Increase the percentage of clients receiving twice yearly educational sessions on CVD prevention and risk reduction to 95% by the end of year 2.

We have reduced the example case study to focus on hypertension. In reality, there would be objectives that addressed other risk factors for CVD as well, such as overwight/obesity, smoking, diabetes, etc.

Southern Primary HealthCare Clinics CVDPC **outcome** objectives:

- Increase by 30% the number of hypertensive clients who have reduced their blood pressure by 13 points after being enrolled in the CVDPC Program for 12 months.
- Increase by 40% the number of hypertensive clients who have achieved normal blood pressure (Systolic <120 and Diastolic <80 mmHg) after being enrolled in the CVDPC program for 24 months.

Objectives provide the focus for your evaluation. Poorly written objectives can lead to confusion over how to collect data or how to interpret results. A good objective is SMART: **S**pecific, **M**easurable, **A**ttainable, **R**elated to goal, and **T**ime-bound.

- **Specific**—clearly defines an event or outcome that will be achieved, with details about time, place and persons
- **Measurable**—defines the level or magnitude of change expected
- **Attainable**—states an ambitious but realistic outcome given available resources
- **Related to goal**—the outcome fits into the broader context of the program and can directly affect the overall program goal
- **Time-bound**—states the timeframe in which the outcome is expected to be achieved

---

It's tempting to want to include many objectives in your first evaluation. It is best to keep your first evaluation fairly small, however, to make sure you can get good results. Only then will your staff be motivated to continue building your evaluation efforts in the future.

Stakeholders should also be involved in developing the list of goals and objectives. If an important stakeholder has a completely different idea about what your program should accomplish, and none of the goals or objectives address that viewpoint, then the stakeholder may not value the evaluation results. Having a meeting with key people to brainstorm objectives can be a quick and efficient way of involving stakeholders.

> Stakeholder input is critical to gaining support for your evaluation and ensuring that the results will be used. But remember that this is **your** evaluation. Do not let competing stakeholder interests overwhelm your evaluation efforts. Remember that the people on your evaluation team are your **most** important stakeholders in the evaluation!

Following are some examples of poorly written outcome objectives, along with improved examples.

	POOR objectives	IMPROVED objectives
Not specific!	Increase the percentage of clients who have learned about better diets to 40% by the end of year 1 of the program.	Increase the percentage of clients who are able to demonstrate knowledge of at least three new low-fat recipes to 40% by the end of year 1 of the program.
Not measurable!	Increase the percentage of CVDPC participants who have learned a lot about CVD by the end of each educational session.	Increase the percentage of CVDPC participants who are able to correctly name risk factors for and ways to prevent CVD by the end of each educational session.
Not attainable!	Increase by 100% the number of hypertensive clients who have achieved normal blood pressure (Systolic <120 and Diastolic <80 mmHg) after being enrolled in the CVDPC program for 24 months.	Increase by 40% the number of hypertensive clients who have achieved normal blood pressure (Systolic <120 and Diastolic <80 mmHg) after being enrolled in the CVDPC program for 24 months.
Not related to goal!	Decrease the percentage of CVDPC participants who are unhappy with their weight by 40% by the end of year 1.	Increase by 40% the percentage of CVDPC participants who have achieved a weight goal set by their physician after 12 months of the program.
Not time-bound!	Increase by 30% the number of hypertensive clients who have reduced their blood pressure by 13 points.	Increase by 30% the number of hypertensive clients who have reduced their blood pressure by 13 points after being enrolled in the CVDPC Program for 12 months.

Refer to the goals and objectives worksheet to fill in your own program objectives. Apply the SMART test to each one to ensure that you have well-written objectives. Then prioritize the objectives by their importance to the overall goal of the program.

You may want to involve your stakeholders in this process, or this may be a step your evaluation team will have to complete on its own (if time is short or if the key stakeholders tend to have a difficult time reaching an agreement). In the end, it is up to your evaluation team to decide what input from stakeholders will be part of the evaluation.

Southern Primary HealthCare Clinics

Objective	Specific?	Measurable?	Attainable?	Related to goal?	Time-bound?	Priority (importance to goal) H- High M-Moderate L- Low
Increase the percentage of clients who are able to demonstrate knowledge of new low-fat recipes to 40% by the end of year 1 of the program.	✓	✓	✓	?	✓	L
Increase the percentage of CVDPC participants who are able to correctly name risk factors for and ways to prevent CVD by the end of each educational session.	✓	✓	✓	✓	✓	M
Increase by 40% the number of hypertensive clients who have achieved normal blood pressure (Systolic <120 and Diastolic <80 mmHg) after being enrolled in the CVDPC program for 24 months.	✓	✓	✓	✓	✓	H
Increase by 40% the percentage of CVDPC participants who have achieved a weight goal set by their physician after 12 months of the program.	✓	✓	✓	✓	✓	L
Increase by 30% the number of hypertensive clients who have reduced their blood pressure by 13 points after being enrolled in the CVDPC Program for 12 months.	✓	✓	✓	✓	✓	H

Develop a Conceptual Framework

Next you will want to lay out your ideas for how the program is expected to achieve its goal, step by step. This is done through developing a conceptual framework. **A conceptual framework shows the sequence of events that are thought to occur in order to bring about the desired changes in the community.**

The conceptual framework diagram, once finished, can then be "read" by following the arrows in order to get the story of how your program is working.

The framework can be completed in any order, the steps given in this section outline just one approach you could take. Your whole evaluation team should be involved in brainstorming the conceptual framework.

Figure 2.3 shows how a blank conceptual framework, to measure the effect of your program activities, looks:

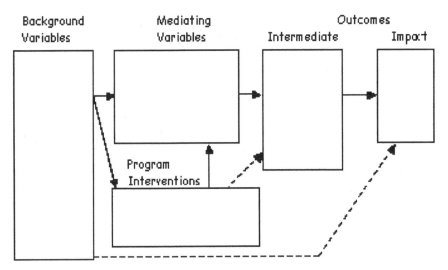

Fig. 2.3 Conceptual Framework for measuring program effectiveness

A Conceptual Framework Consists of Five Basic Components:

- Background variables—these are aspects of the target population (age, sex, education, socio-demographics, past health history, etc.) that are not altered by the program intervention but that may influence a person's access to the program.
- Mediating Variables—these are aspects of your target population such as their knowledge, attitudes, or beliefs.
- Intervention—these are the activities that your program will carry out to achieve its goals and objectives.
- Intermediate outcomes—these are behaviors of the target population that your intervention is trying to change.
- Long-term outcomes (impact)—these are the eventual effects that your program hopes to achieve, usually measured in terms of a biological change (e.g., blood pressure).

You will note from the conceptual framework diagram that there is actually more than one way for the final outcome to be reached.

> Some people will have negative outcomes regardless of how well your program works, so you should never list a goal of '100%' improvement.

- Background variables alone can determine the outcome. For example, "family history of heart disease" could directly lead to an outcome of heart disease in a person despite any change in mediating variables if the cause of disease was mostly genetic. This means that, even if a program addressing heart disease were to succeed in getting 100% of the population to completely eliminate all behavioral risk factors, it still could not eliminate heart disease.

- There is a pathway from background variables through mediating variables and to outcomes that doesn't go through the program intervention at all. Some of the target population will achieve changes in mediating variables, intermediate and final outcomes even without a program intervention. In the heart disease example, some at-risk people might decide to start exercising more and adopt a healthier diet even without the benefit of the program interventions.

The items you fill in on your conceptual framework are exactly those items that you will collect information on. For example, if you fill in a mediating variable of "Believes that HIV can be prevented," you will later need to determine some way of measuring this among your participants.

> Use the 'Developing a conceptual framework' worksheet in page 148 to create your own conceptual framework.

In order to measure the long-term outcomes, it is necessary to gather information at two different time points for the same individual. The first time point should always be at the very start of your program, before those individuals have had any contact with your services (baseline). Only in this way can you show the changes among your participants after having utilized your services.

Just as the name implies, "long-term outcomes" happen over a long period of time. You will probably not be able to measure changes in the long-term impact on your first evaluation. Instead, you will want to measure changes in behaviors—the intermediate outcomes. Later, you can go back and see if changes in the intermediate outcomes truly led to changes in the long-term outcomes for your participants.

On the next page Fig. 2.4 shows an example of what a completed conceptual framework might look like.

Define Methodological Approach for Evaluation

The strongest type of evaluation is one that uses an **experimental design.** In an experimental design, the target population is separated into two groups. The first group receives the program interventions you have developed, the second group does not. Assignment of people into the two groups is made randomly, just as if you had flipped a coin to decide. At the end of some period of time, you observe the

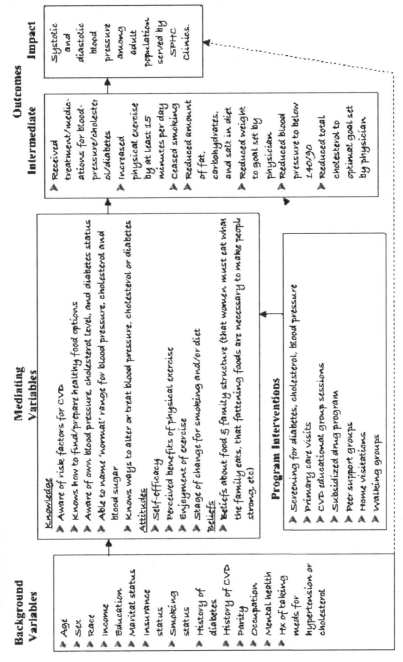

Conceptual framework for measuring change in blood pressure among clients who are enrolled in the CVDPC

Background Variables

- Age
- Sex
- Race
- Income
- Education
- Marital status
- Insurance status
- Smoking status
- History of diabetes
- History of CVD
- Parity
- Occupation
- Mental health
- Hx of taking meds for hypertension or cholesterol

Mediating Variables

Knowledge
- Aware of risk factors for CVD
- Knows how to find/prepare healthy food options
- Aware of own blood pressure, cholesterol level, and diabetes status
- Able to name 'normal' range for blood pressure, cholesterol and blood sugar
- Knows ways to alter or treat blood pressure, cholesterol or diabetes

Attitudes
- Self-efficacy
- Perceived benefits of physical exercise
- Enjoyment of exercise
- Stage of change for smoking and/or diet

Beliefs
- Beliefs about food & family structure (that women must eat what the family eats, that fattening foods are necessary to make people strong, etc)

Program Interventions

- Screening for diabetes, cholesterol, blood pressure
- Primary care visits
- CVD educational group sessions
- Subsidized drug program
- Peer support groups
- Home visitations
- Walking groups

Outcomes

Intermediate

- Received treatment/medications for blood pressure/cholesterol/diabetes
- Increased physical exercise by at least 15 minutes per day
- Ceased smoking
- Reduced amount of fat, carbohydrates, and salt in diet
- Reduced weight to goal set by physician
- Reduced blood pressure to below 140/90
- Reduced total cholesterol to optimal goal set by physician

Impact

- Systolic and diastolic blood pressure among adult population served by SPHC Clinics.

Fig. 2.4

two groups and see if the group that received the intervention had better health outcomes than the group that did not. Although experimental designs are the most convincing, they can be rather complicated and are therefore not as common as other designs.

Strengths of an experimental design:

- Can show that changes are really due to your intervention, and not other factors.

It is almost never ethical to deny services to one group of people in order to compare them to another group that receives services. Instead, when conducting an experimental design, you may decide to provide expanded or different services to one group, while maintaining the normal level of services for another group in order to see if the changes introduced by the expanded services were beneficial.

Problems with experimental designs include:

- Random assignment takes extra time and effort. It might also not be possible to truly divide people up randomly.
- Random assignment can cause ethical concerns. For example, if running a dental clinic in a school, it would probably not be ethical to offer free dental care to only half the children who needed it.

An alternative to the experimental design is the **quasi-experimental** design. "Quasi" means *as if* or *almost*, so a quasi-experimental design is "almost-experimental." In these types of evaluation, there are again two groups that are compared, except assignment to one group or the other is not random. For example, if conducting an educational session in a school, one classroom may get the session while the other does not. Because students were not assigned randomly, however (they were assigned based on which class they were in), it can be difficult to determine if there were other differences between the classes that was really responsible for any changes seen. Perhaps one class had a more dynamic teacher, or brighter students, or a better atmosphere of communication and collaboration than the other class.

Another form of quasi-experimental design that is quite common is the pretest-posttest design. In this kind of evaluation, participants are surveyed before they engage in the program activities on their knowledge, beliefs, etc. Then, after a set amount of time of participation in the program, they are surveyed again. The results of the later time period are compared to the beginning time period to see if any changes occurred. The benefit of this type of design is that there is no need for a comparison group—participants serve as their own comparison. The drawbacks are the same as any quasi-experimental design, in that you cannot be absolutely sure that the program caused the changes observed.

> **Bias:** refers to some factor that distorts the truth or causes you to reach conclusions that are not correct.
>
> **Example:** You ask physicians to recommend clients for a new counseling service. You compare the mental health improvements in the clients enrolled in the program to those who were not, and conclude that the program worked in helping people improve their mental health. But the physicians recommended mostly those clients who were compliant, friendly, and already improving. So your results are biased.
>
> **Some other factors – in this case:** the selection of clients who were already improving – explains why that group did better than the non-enrolled group, not your program intervention.

The most common evaluation design is **observational**. It is the easiest to perform, as participants are not divided or randomized into groups of any sort. You simply *observe* what happens as participants interact with your program and then report on the results. The drawback of this design is that there is often a good deal of *bias* involved, which makes the results less convincing.

To summarize:

- Experimental designs can show that changes in the population were the result of the program.
- Quasi-experimental designs can *suggest* that the changes were a result of the program. Observational designs can only show that the program was *associated* with a change in the population, which may have resulted from the program or may have resulted in some other factors.
- Consider the following example of an experimental, quasi-experimental, and observational design for the same program intervention.

> **Southern Primary HealthCare Clinics**
>
> Experimental design
> Southern Primary Health (SPHC) Clinics instructed their physicians that every other client who came to the clinic that was identified as being at risk for CVD were to be enrolled in their new CVDPC program. After assignment to the two groups was finished, the group receiving the new program services were very similar to the group that did not. The average age, body-mass index, blood pressure, cholesterol level, and fat intake were all nearly the same between the two groups, as were smoking status, diabetic status, insurance status, and other key variables.

Because the only real known difference between the 2 groups was the CVDPC program services, the fact that the CVDPC group had much greater improvements in blood pressure y at the end of 2 years was taken as evidence that the program caused the improvements in blood pressure.

Quasi-experimental design
SPHC Clinics decided to offer their expanded CVD prevention and Control program to all of their at-risk clients at 1 of their clinics, but not to the at-risk clients at their second clinic in the same county. A pretest given to all clients at both clinics showed that levels of knowledge about CVD were similar at both. Clients at the intervention clinic had slightly worse health than those at the 'control' clinic, though. At the end of 2 years, 20% of patients at the intervention clinics had achieved normal blood pressure, while only 12% of patients at the control clinic had.

The conclusion was that the program appeared to lead to improvements in blood pressure. There was no way to tell, however, whether perhaps the physicians at one clinic were more engaged than the other, whether the clients at one clinic differed in important ways (such as income, insurance status, motivation to improve health, feelings of self-efficacy, etc), or whether there were other important differences between the clinic environments that could have influenced the results.

Observational design
SPHS offered its new CVDPC program to all of its high-risk clients at all of its clinics. Some clients enrolled, while others declined to participate. At the end of the 2 years, the clinics compared those clients who enrolled to those that didn't. They also compared the overall CVD rate before the program to the rate after 2 years of the program. Clients enrolled in the program had a lower rate of CVD than those not enrolled, and the overall rate had dropped over the 2 years. Also, 20% of clients enrolled in the program had achieved normal blood pressure after 2 years, while only 10% of other at-risk SPHS clients had achieved normal blood pressure over the same time period.

The conclusion was that the program seemed to be associated with a decrease in CVD. Questions that could not be answered included: did only the lower-risk clients sign up for the program, while the higher risk group – who would normally have a higher rate of CVD – decline (explaining the difference between groups)? Was there a general trend in the population towards lower CVD rates over the 2 years of the program (explaining the difference over time)? Were those that signed up for the program already working towards improving their blood pressure, so that the difference would have existed even had the program never existed? These questions reflect the fact that the findings may not be 'real' – there may be bias (other factors that explain the differences between the groups).

Select Indicators

Before you can start planning how to collect data for your evaluation, you have to decide exactly what information you need to collect. Once you have your program goals and objectives outlined, and have a conceptual framework to better visualize the program, decide on indicators to guide the data collection. **Indicators are ways of measuring changes related to your objectives and program activities.** Often, there will need to be more than one indicator for a single objective.

> Whenever possible, you should use established indicators already in use by the census bureau or other organizations working in your field. This makes it easier for others to understand exactly what changes your program is creating. The reference list at the back of the book gives some resources to find already established indicators.

For some objectives, the indicators will be very easy and straightforward. For example, if one objective is "at the end of the first year of the program, 90% of children at School X will be fully vaccinated," then a sensible indicator for the objective would be "the percent of children at School X who are fully vaccinated." The indicator is the actual measurement you will use to assess changes related to the objective.

It is very important not to change your indicators over time. You want to be able to compare your results from one time period to another, but you won't be able to make such a comparison if your indicators were different at the two time points.

Prioritizing Indicators

Collecting data on indicators takes time and resources. If your list of indicators is pretty long, you may not be able to address them all in your first evaluation. Prioritize based on importance to evaluation and ease of measurement.

Develop a Data Collection and Analysis Plan

Once you have your list of objectives and indicators, you will have to decide on the best way to collect and analyze the data. A carefully detailed plan will save you many headaches and frustrations further down the road.

Southern Primary HealthCare Clinics

Objective	Priority (Importance to **goal**) H-High M-Moderate L-Low	Indicators for objective	Ease of data collection 0-Data already available 1-easy to collect 2-possible 3- difficult	Priority of indicator 1-Critical to <u>objective</u> 2-Important 3-Can do without	Overall score (H,M, or L – and sum of previous 2 columns Ex: *M-1*)
Increase the percentage of clients who are able to demonstrate knowledge of at least three new low-fat recipes to 40% by the end of year 1 of the program.	L	Pre-post questions #10,11 & 12 on client questionnaire	1	2	L-3
		Score of 10 or above in cooking demonstration session	2	2	L-4
Increase the percentage of CVDPC participants who are able to correctly name risk factors for and ways to prevent CVD by the end of the educational session.	M	Pre-post questions #5, 6 & 7 on client questionnaire	1	1	M-2
Increase by 40% the number of hypertensive clients who have achieved normal blood pressure (Systolic <120 and Diastolic <80mmHg) after being enrolled in the CVDPC program for 24 months.	H	Blood pressure at or below 120mmHg systolic and 80mmHg diastolic	1	1	H-2
Increase by 40% the percentage of CVDPC participants who have achieved a weight goal set by their physician after 12 months of the program.	L	Weight is at or below goal set in clinic records by physician	1	1	L-2
Increase by 30% the number of hypertensive clients who have reduced their blood pressure by 13 points after being enrolled in the CVDPC Program for 12 months.	H	Systolic blood pressure measurement	1	1	H-2

First, take stock of what information is already out there and available. With your list of indicators on hand, consider the following possible data sources and determine if any of them may provide you with enough information to satisfy your indicators:

- ❑ Your own logs & records
- ❑ Client medical records
- ❑ County vital records
- ❑ Client satisfaction surveys

- ❑ Census data
- ❑ Service statistics
- ❑ Intercept questionnaires
- ❑ Inventory logs

> Using a little of both qualitative and quantitative methods is the best way to go! Quantitative tells you 'how much' and qualitative tells you 'why' or 'how'. Together, they give you the full story!

If you need to collect additional information, there are two basic types of data collection methods that you can choose from: qualitative and quantitative. Qualitative data are used for explanatory purposes; they aim to *describe* something. Quantitative data are number-based; they are *counts* of something.

Examples	Used for	Strengths	Weaknesses
QUALITATIVE			
• Interviews • Case Studies • Observations • Journals or diaries • Open-ended survey questions	• Answer the question *why* • Discover ideas, perceptions, feelings, or beliefs • Explore a poorly understood subject • Explains and adds depth to quantitative data	• Open-ended can explore even poorly understood topics • Gives details, context, & "depth"	• Analysis of data can be difficult • Requires more staff and participant time • Cannot answer how large or widespread an issue is • May not apply to entire population (data collected from relatively few individuals)

Examples	Used for	Strengths	Weaknesses
QUANTITATIVE			
• Surveys • Knowledge tests • Activity logs • Clinical records	• Answer the questions "how much" or "how many" • Can be used to compare against other data, statistics, or indicators • Looking at relationships between factors using statistical analysis	• Large number of participants— "wider" data more applicable to full population • Structured methods • Analysis and interpretation easier	• Information restricted to what is asked, cannot explore topics or perspectives outside of standardized questions • Does not provide a context for the data

Along with the method of data collection, decide on the *timing* of collection. For process evaluations, some forms of data collection (logs, diaries, attendance sheets, etc.) will probably be ongoing, while others (interviews, discussion groups, etc.) will be done only periodically. For outcome evaluations, you will want to establish a baseline if the program is just beginning. Whatever stage the project is in, you may need to collect data more than once.

> Take care when establishing a baseline, as information left out at the beginning will limit what you are able to compare later on.

Consider the following:

- Does seasonality influence who uses your program or what the likely results would be? For example, a school-based program may have very different clients in the summer than in the winter.
- Do you serve a stable population base, or do clients rotate through the program often? For programs in which clients come and go frequently, you may want to collect data at several points to capture the range of clients served.
- How quickly do you expect change to occur among those served by your program? If your program focuses on long-term effects, such as stable weight loss, it may be best to space out data collection efforts by a significant (1–2 years) time frame.

> Follow the conceptual framework that you developed and think about how long you expect certain outcomes to take to be achieved.
>
> If you collect data too early, it may look like your program is having no effect when in reality it is simply taking longer for changes to occur.
>
> If you wait too long to collect data you may miss important changes in the population, and it may be more difficult to determine exactly how the program worked.

Data Base Creation

Whichever method(s) of data collection you choose for your evaluation, you must have some system in place for storing and organizing the data if it is to be used to monitor or evaluate the program.

> Chapter 4 and Appendices 1 (data collection tools) and 2 (worksheet) provide more information on database creation and data entry.

For any sort of quantitative data, this means establishing a *database*. There are many software programs that you could use to create your own database, including:

- Epi Info
- CSPro
- Microsoft Excel
- Filemaker Pro
- Microsoft Access

If your project already has a database set up, it may be best to stick with the same system. Most programs allow the data to be exported into different formats. If your program does not have the capacity to do data analysis and create charts and figures, an option may be to export the data to one of the free programs (such as Epi Info) for that purpose.

A database is an organized collection of information that is stored in such a way as to allow for easy access and analysis.

Qualitative data is a bit trickier to deal with. It is really just words, comments, and stories, which may not be easily grouped or analyzed. For storing qualitative data, you need a word processing program, such as Microsoft Word, Word Perfect, or even just a text editor that comes free on most computers. "Entering the data" means simply typing out the interviews, case studies or discussions into the word processor.

Analyzing qualitative data requires different types of software, such as NUD*IST, Xsight, The Ethnograph, and Atlas/TI, but these are complex and take a while to learn.

The Centers for Disease Control and prevention have a free software package available, called EZ-Text, that may be easier than most. The important thing to make sure of before beginning qualitative data collection is that you have some sort of word processing program and at least one staff member who is a good typist and will be able to spend some time after each data collection to transcribe the information.

CDC software for quantitative (Epi Info) and qualitative (EZ-Text) data are free and easy to use. Instruction guides and tutorials are also available.
The websites for these programs are:
Epi Info: http://www.cdc.gov/epiinfo
EZ-Text: http://www.cdc.gov/hiv/software/ez-text.htm

Lastly, develop a plan for backing up and storing any databases or files you create during the evaluation. Imagine going through all the effort of conducting a survey, entering the data, and analyzing the information to have the computer crash and take all your hard work with it! Some ways to back up data include:

- Saving it to a central server
- Zip drives
- External hard-drive

It is also a good idea to store back-ups in a different building or location, in the unlikely event of a fire or catastrophic event. Your data is precious, so these simple and inexpensive steps are something to seriously consider!

Mock Tables

A good way to determine if you have are on the right track with your data collection plan is to draft mock tables. What do you want to show at the end of your evaluation? What do your ideal tables or diagrams look like? Draft up some imaginary tables that you would like to see at the end of the evaluation, and then go back through your data collection plan to determine whether you think it is able to produce what you want.

Chapter 4 will have more information on creating mock tables

Ethics and Confidentiality

Another key aspect to consider during the planning stages of the evaluation is confidentiality. In order for your evaluation to meet ethical standards, you must have a system for protecting the safety and privacy of all the people who will contribute information.
Aspects of ethical conduct that need to be considered include:

- **Informed consent.** All participants in your evaluation must be told what the evaluation is all about, how you will use the information, whether they will be identified, and that they can refuse to participate with no repercussions.

See chapter 3 for more information on ethics and confidentiality in data collection

- **Confidentiality**. This applies to several stages of the evaluation.
  - *During the data collection.*
  - *During data entering/storage.*
  - *When reporting the results*
- **Safety and well-being**. This includes both physical and mental/emotional safety of people who may participate in your evaluation and of your own staff.

If you plan to publish any part of your evaluation results, you may need to consider getting an IRB (Institutional Review Board) to review and approve your evaluation plan in advance. Most hospitals and universities have their own IRBs, which are often willing to review and approve plans from community organizations. Having IRB approval will help assure that your evaluation is planned in an ethical manner, and will make it easier to use and distribute your evaluation results.

Plan for Dissemination of Evaluation Results

The last part of your evaluation plan should be in preparation for how to disseminate and use the results. All of the stakeholders you named earlier in the evaluation plan are potential audiences for the evaluation results.

> An Institutional Review Board is a group of professionals who review and approve plans for research studies – including evaluations. This is done to protect participants in the study or evaluation.
> Each IRB will likely have a different application process and deadlines – so ask early if you think you will need IRB approval.

Stakeholders don't all need the same types or amount of information from your evaluation. Other community health groups will likely desire the most amount of information from your program, including performance measures and outcomes.

Politicians, on the other hand, probably don't need much information on implementation, and community members probably aren't that concerned with the amount of resources used. Plan ahead with your stakeholders to determine what they are interested in and what information needs to be shared with them after the evaluation.

Information dissemination should not wait until after the evaluation is finished. Keep stakeholders engaged in the evaluation process by providing regular reports. A good option may be to schedule periodic meetings with stakeholders, during which you can offer information and solicit feedback from them during the same time frame.

There are many different formats that you could choose to present information about your evaluation, whether giving periodic updates or presenting a final report. Planning ahead will help you ensure you collect the necessary materials for dissemination later.

- Written report
- Oral presentation
- Newsletter
- Press release or newspaper article
- Visual presentation

You will likely want to use a combination of the presentation methods, as different audiences respond to different formats. It is worthwhile to invest in a communication plan. Evaluation results can be great publicity for your program, helping you to gain more funding, obtain additional support from communities and political leaders, and build relationships with other community groups.

> More information on the use and dissemination of evaluation results is provided in chapter 5.

As part of the plan, you should also determine how you will *use* the results of the evaluation. Will the results be used to gain more funding? To advocate for policy changes on a local or state level? To gain support from community members or other organizations? In all cases, the results should be used to improve and enhance your own program, and to provide some accountability to donors and the people your program serves.

Once you have a plan for your evaluation in place, you can move on to the next step-collecting data.

Chapter 2 checklist—Operationalize the Evaluation Plan

- ❑ Evaluation team selected
- ❑ Review of program target, program description
- ❑ Goals and objectives defined
- ❑ Conceptual framework developed
- ❑ Selected study design for evaluation
- ❑ Indicators selected and prioritized
- ❑ Data collection and analysis plan complete
- ❑ Plan for the dissemination and use of evaluation results

Chapter 3
Obtain Data

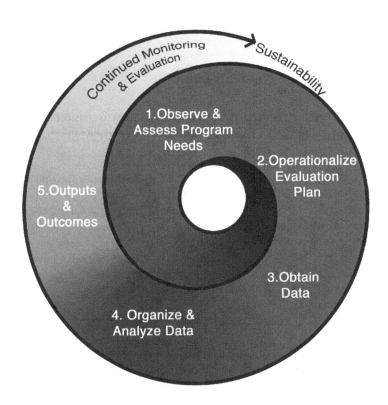

Contents

Obtain Data

This chapter provides more details on how to collect data for your evaluation. Beyond just gathering information, data collection entails considerations of ethics and confidentiality, data storage, and data quality. By the end of this chapter you should have a better idea of how to appropriately collect information for your evaluation.

> Although data storage and database creation are covered in chapter 4, it may be helpful for you to review that section before beginning data collection to ensure that you will be able to appropriately store the data you collect.

Ethical Conduct & Confidentiality

Before you even begin to plan your data collection, you need to consider how you will protect the rights and privacy of people from whom you will gather information.

> It is very, very rare that the benefits of not telling participants the true intent of your evaluation could outweigh the harms. An example of a situation where it might be OK would be if you were conducting a survey to see if physicians treat patients differently based on their race or gender. In that case, telling the physicians the true question you are trying to answer would likely influence their answers. In almost all situations that Community Health Care organizations encounter, however, the negative consequences and ethical problems of misleading participants will outweigh any benefit to your evaluation.

'Ethical conduct' in data collection includes:

- **Being open and honest with study participants**. In very rare circumstances, it is OK to be vague about some aspect of the evaluation (usually when knowing more details could alter people's responses), but it is **never** OK to deceive or mislead participants. **Deceiving or misleading participants includes omitting information, as well as giving wrong information.**
- **Protecting the safety of the participants**. This includes ensuring that participants are not subject to undue stress, embarrassment, physical or emotional pain, anxiety, or other harm.
- **Ensuring that participants are not coerced or led into saying or doing something**. Participation in an evaluation activity must be entirely voluntary. Coercion would include actions such as threatening to reduce services if a person did not participate, pleading or badgering a person, or attempting to

make a person feel guilty for not participating. It also includes offering incentives for participating that are so high a person will participate because they feel they can't afford to refuse. Leading a participant into saying something can also occur during the evaluation, by asking leading questions during a group interview or on a survey.

- **Assuring confidentiality of participants.** This is exceptionally important during an evaluation. Names of participants must never be used in reports or made public in any way. Even within your project, only a very small number of people should have access to any records you may keep of who participated in an evaluation activity (it is usually best to destroy all records with names, unless you will need them for follow-up or some other justified purpose).

You need to be careful that your data cannot be traced back to individual participants, even if you have removed names. For example, there may only be one Hispanic pediatrician in her 50s living in a certain community – including just that much information will identify her as surely as including her name!

Informed Consent

You should obtain **informed consent** from any person that you would like to recruit for an evaluation activity. Informed consent means just what it says—that a person consents to participate after being properly informed about what is involved. To 'properly inform' someone, you need to tell them (at minimum):

- Who is conducting the data collection
- The purpose of the data collection
- Why they were chosen to be included
- How the information collected will be used
- What the benefits and risks are to people who consent to participate
- How confidentiality will be assured
- A statement on how they can change their mind about participating at any time
- Who they should contact to have any questions answered

After explaining the above points to a would-be participant, the person gives his or her consent. Most often consent is given by signing an informed consent form, a copy of which you keep for your records and a copy of which you give to the participant to keep. In some cases, such as a telephone survey, informed consent can be verbal. In both cases, however, you should have an informed consent form that you can read off of, to make sure you cover all the relevant information.

Examples of informed consent forms are in Appendix 2, pp. 153.

Even if you believe your questions are easy and not likely to embarrass someone or cause any problems, you still need to be careful to protect the confidentiality of your participants. You never know what may be sensitive to a particular person. Also, if your clients or community members see that you are not careful about keeping their answers or information private, they may be less likely to give honest answers or to be willing to answer sensitive questions in the future.

> Informed consent can be difficult with populations who cannot reasonably give informed consent, such as mentally disabled persons or young children. In those cases, you should get the consent of a guardian or parent as well. The participant should still have the activity explained to them in the best way possible, and be asked if they agree to participate, but the guardian or parent would need to actually sign the informed consent form.

Ensuring ethical conduct

Consider forming a **Community Advisory Board (CAB)** for your evaluation. Ask five–six community members who can represent the population you will involve in your evaluation to volunteer to review your evaluation questions, informed consent process, and protections of confidentiality. Ask the CAB for their opinion on whether certain questions may be too sensitive or confusing, and whether your informed consent is likely to be understood by most of your participants.

> Institutional Review Board (IRB) approval is also a good way to ensure that you have taken the proper steps to protect your participants, in addition to pilot testing and having a Community Advisory Board.

Pilot test any data collection questions you will use on a small number (usually five–ten) of people from the population who will participate in the evaluation. Check to see what may have been confusing or uncomfortable for them, and ask them questions afterwards to see if they understood the consent form and how they felt about participating.

Qualitative Versus Quantitative Methods

In Chapter 2, you were given some guidance on how to develop and prioritize indicators for your evaluation. In order to decide the best way to collect data on your indicators, these are some questions you could ask:

- Does the indicator address a topic that is not well understood? (e.g. people's beliefs or perceptions).
- Is the purpose of the data collection to provide a deeper understanding of an issue (such as 'how' or 'why')?
- Is it important that participants be able to give their own perspectives and feedback?

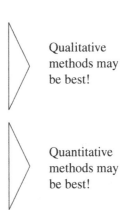

Qualitative methods may be best!

- Is the purpose of the data collection to figure out how widespread an issue is, or how many people it affects?
- Do you want to use the data to make a statement about a larger group of people (including those that did not directly give information)?
- Is it important that you be able to give figures and tables to donors or stakeholders

Quantitative methods may be best!

It is possible, and in fact beneficial, to include both qualitative and quantitative methods in your evaluation. Qualitative is usually used to inform your quantitative methods, or to 'fill out' or explain the quantitative results. A few of the more common ways of collecting either type of information are explained below.

Qualitative Data Collection Methods

In-depth Interviews

- Brief description:
    - A single person (often called a 'key informant') is asked about a particular topic during a face-to-face discussion with a member of your evaluation team (or some other trained person).
    - There is not a rigid set of questions. Instead, the interviewer tries to have the respondent answer at length about fewer, broader questions, and encourages the respondent to give information that does not exactly follow the questions.

> When done properly, in-depth interviews should flow like a casual conversation between two people (except with the respondent doing most of the talking!).

- When it is used:
    - When you believe that a certain person or set of people have particularly relevant opinions or information that you think would be better explored in a one-on-one situation.
    - Can help you form questions for group interviews or surveys to be held later, or can replace group interviews when the subject is too sensitive for people to respond in a group situation.

> In-depth interviews can last anywhere from 30 min to 2 h, depending on the number of questions you have and how in depth you want to go.

- Strengths:
  - Can help you explore a new area or an issue that you don't understand well yet
  - Useful for understanding the reasoning or emotions of participants (gives the 'full story')
- Weaknesses:
  - Time burden is high for staff and participants
  - Can be difficult to figure out what to do with information collected

Group Interviews

- Brief description:
  - Semi-structured group discussions that involve anywhere from 6 to 12 people. A trained group facilitator asks the questions that the group is to answer, and ensures that the conversation doesn't stray too far from the 'focus' of the group.
  - Allows respondents to listen to other people's responses, and contribute to the discussion themselves.

> Group interviews are also called 'focus groups'. This manual will not cover all the various details of how to do full focus group procedures. In order to differentiate this shortened version from the full version, we call the technique a 'group interview', rather than a 'focus group'. If you are interested in performing a full focus group, there are resoures that you can look up in the reference list at the end of this book.

- When used:
  - When you want a deeper understanding of the feelings, thoughts, and opinions of the population from which the group participants were selected.
- Strengths:
  - Can bring out opinions and insights that would not otherwise appear on single interviews.
  - Good way of getting information to guide the development of a survey or other questionnaire
- Weaknesses:
  - Confidentiality issues can be a problem (cannot guarantee that others in the group will not speak about what is said outside of the room)

- Require a good deal of time from staff members to transcribe information
- Sometimes so much information is gained it can be difficult to know how to sort or use it.

Case studies

- Brief description:
    - A detailed description of the experience of a single person, instance, or group. Reads like a story of what happened.

> Case studies are basically just stories of what happened, with many different points of view represented and the highest level of accuracy possible. They are useful in evaluation as they are highly readable, usually very interesting, and allow the reader to "walk through" the experience of whomever or whatever the cast study is about.

- When used:
    - They are most often used when a project is new or unique (to better understand how the program impacts the people it serves) or to highlight aspects of a survey or other evaluation data (to make the data more understandable and 'human').
- Strengths:
    - Can reveal details about an activity or program that were overlooked
    - Gives a 'personal' touch, can be more interesting to reader
- Weaknesses:
    - High time commitment from staff and sometimes participants
    - Can be difficult to pick the focus (person or object)
    - Confidentiality can be a problem

Observations

- Brief description:
    - When a member of the evaluation team watches an event or activity and records what happens.

> Be sure to consider whether the presence of an observer will affect the situation being observed. If observing a client interacting with a nurse, for instance, are both more likely to be nicer and more professional due to the observer being in the room?

- When used:
  - You want to fully understand the details of how an event or occurrence happens. Examples might be:
    - → Client's visit with a case worker, nurse, or other program staff may be observed to more fully understand the dynamics of the interactions;
    - → An educational seminar may be observed to understand the dynamics of the sessions, the skill and demeanor of the educator, and the reactions of the participants;
    - → Members of the community may be observed in their own homes, offices, schools, etc. to get a clearer idea of situations of interest to the program.
  - You want to obtain more accurate information than you may otherwise get by asking people in a questionnaire or interview. For instance,
    - → Observing a client performing a certain task could give more accurate information than asking the client how they perform the task;
    - → Observing people interact could provide a better understanding than asking the people themselves (examples could be a parent and child discussing a dispute, or a group of people in a meeting, etc).
  - When it is an easier option for obtaining information than other data collection methods. For instance,
    - → Observing program staff conduct a client meeting or educational seminar may be easier than questioning the participants to describe the interactions;
    - → Visiting a school, neighborhood, or other location and observing conditions, such as trash, graffiti, etc., could be easier than surveying residents about conditions.
- Strengths:
  - Quick and efficient way to find out how some event happens
  - Can be more accurate than asking others to describe something
- Weaknesses:
  - Limited to events or occurrences that can be directly observed
  - Can be subject to observer's interpretations and attention to detail (two people watching the same event may not notice the same things).

Quantitative Data Collection Methods

End of Session Questionnaires

> Most end-of-session questionnaires are anonymous, allowing respondents to answer more honestly.

- Brief description:
  - A short set of questions that you have everyone who participated in some activity to complete when the activity is over.
  - Purpose may be to obtain feedback on the activity, suggestions for improvement, or to ask about satisfaction, items learned, or skills gained during the activity.
- When used:
  - Can be used after any sort of interaction with your project (such as after an educational seminar, a meeting with a physician, nurse, or case worker, etc)
- Strengths:
  - Cheap and convenient way of getting information
  - Can get information from almost everyone who participates in program activities
- Weaknesses:
  - Participants must be able to read & write in the language of the questionnaire
  - May get poor responses if participants feel rushed, do not feel questionnaire is important, or feel pressured by being at site and around project staff and/or other participants to give positive answers
  - Nearly always anonymous—cannot link participant answers back to other information on that person gathered at another time

Pre-Post Tests
- Brief description:
  - A series of questions given to participants both before and after engaging in some program activity.

> Pre-Post tests are used to determine what may have changed in a participant's knowledge, skills, attitudes, or beliefs as a result of your program activity.

- When used:
  - Used whenever participants will be engaging in an activity that is hoping to teach them some new knowledge or skill, or to change their views or attitudes about a particular topic.
- Strengths:
  - Quick and easy way to determine the immediate effect that the activity has on participants' knowledge, skills, or attitudes.
  - Requires minimal resources and staff time
- Weaknesses:
  - Does not give information on retention of knowledge of attitudes (which may change or be lost after a few weeks or months after the activity)
  - When testing knowledge, administering the pre-test may 'prime' participants so that they do better on the post-test than if they had participated in the activity without having taken a pre-test

Information is generalizable when it can be applied to the full population, even though the information was obtained from only a small number of people from that population. The way to do this is to make the smaller group that is surveyed a reflection of the larger population in terms of important factors such as age, race, gender, economic status, etc.

Surveys

- Brief description:
  - A set of questions given in a standard way to a small group of people chosen to represent a larger group or population of people.
  - The purpose is to gain information that can be generalized to a full population.
- When used:
  - When you want to know about the characteristics of a group of people to plan appropriate interventions, know who is using your services, or measure the effect of your program.
- Strengths:
  - When selection of participants is done well, can provide information about a large group of people by only asking a small subset of that group
  - Usually the best way to information on specific topics from a large number of people
- Weaknesses:
  - High level of resources and staff time often needed.
  - Structured questions do not often leave room for new information that you didn't think to ask.

Basics of Sampling

It is often the case that you can't gather information from *all* of the people that you are interested in hearing from. Instead, you can gather information from a *sample* of the people. As long as that sample is representative of the larger group, you can use their information to make statements about the full group. The process of selecting people to represent the full group is called *sampling*.

"Random" sampling means you pick people in a way that does not follow a pattern or plan, such as by a flip of a coin.

Simple Random Sampling

One way of getting a representative group of people is to do simple **random sample**. The following are examples of how to do a simple random sample:
- Choose numbers out of a hat and ask the people whose client numbers match the ones you draw
  - Get a list of random numbers from the internet (http://www.random.org/nform. html is one site of many that will do this) and select participants whose client IDs match the number generated.

- Benefits of simple random sampling include:
  - It is the best way to get a sample that is not *biased*. Any other type of sampling usually ends up following some sort of pattern that may make your small group different in some way from the larger group it is supposed to represent.
  - It's a more respected method by politicians and others who conduct or are interested in evaluations.

- Problems with simple random sampling include:
  - It requires that you have a list of *all possible* participants to randomly choose from. This may be easy if it's just all of your clients, or it may be very difficult if it's all of the people who live in a certain area.
  - There is no guarantee that the group that is selected will be truly representative of the full population you are interested in. This is especially true when you are selecting just a few people.

Stratified Random Sampling

In stratified random sampling, you do the same thing as you would in a simple random sample. The difference is that you decide ahead of time that you want a certain number of people who have a particular charateristic. The following are two different examples of stratified random sampling:

> Only the very basics of sampling are explained here. Further resources that can help you are listed in the reference list at the end of this book.

- You want to choose six people for a focus group, but because 80% of the population is older a random sample fails to give you any younger people. In stratifed random sampling, you first choose four people at random who are older from all possible older persons, then you choose two people at random who are younger from all possible younger persons.
- You want to compare outcomes among Hispanic persons in your community to Whites, but Hispanics make up only 5% of the population. Rather than a simple

random sample (which would give you around 95 Whites for every 5 Hispanics), do a stratified sampling by first randomly choosing from all Hispanics and then randomly choosing an equal number of Whites from all Whites.
- Benefits of stratified random sampling include:
  - Ensures that you have the representation you want of certain kinds of people
  - Can increase the efficiency of your data collection by providing the 'optimal' distribution of the characteristic of interest.
- Problems with stratified random sampling include:
  - It requires more effort than simple random sampling (you have to do multiple random samples)

Systematic Random Sampling

Again similar to simple random sampling, except that you choose every second person, or every third person, etc. from a list. For example, if you have a list of 1,000 clients, and you want to survey 100, you would choose every tenth client from the list.

> Divide the total number of possible participants by the number you want to include to get the interval between selections. If you want 100 clients out of 900 possible, then you would choose every $1000 \div 900 = $ 9th person.

- Benefits of systematic random sampling include:
  - Very simple and easy to implement
  - Can be adapted for use without having a full list of all possible participants. For example, you can tell your clinicians to interview every fifth person who walks through the door.
- Problems with systematic random sampling include:
  - There may be patterns inherent in the list that you are using that would make your sample differ in some systematic way from the rest of the population. This is especially true if you are simply picking every *nth* person who walks through the door (example—if you average five clients a day and you always pick the fifth, you will always get people who come late in the day, who may be different from those who come early).

Purposive Sampling

Purposive sampling is when you select people on purpose—based on who they are and what you already know about them. This is generally used only for qualitative methods.

Non-random sampling methods (purposive and convenience) should be used with caution, and are usually only useful for qualitative data methods. This is because they almost never give you a representative sample.

Examples of purposive sampling might include:

- You want to find out more information from clients who voiced complaints about your program so you ask those clients
- You invite certain community leaders who you know have a great deal of influence over others in the community
- Benefits of purposive sampling include:
  - Very simple and convenient way of hearing from the people you want to hear from.
- Problems with purposive sampling include:
  - It is not a random sample. Your sample will be a *biased* sample of the full population, and should not be used to generalize.

Convenience Sample

A more common way of selecting participants is to gather a **convenience sample**. This means that you ask whoever happens to be around at the time that you want to hold the group. For example, you may ask all the clients who walk into a clinic on a particular afternoon to join the group interview.

Resources that go into more depth on ethics, data collection methods and sampling are listed in the reference list at the end of the book.

- Benefits of convenience sampling include:
  - Requires the least time and resources of any method (hence its name).
- Problems with convenience sampling include:
  - It almost never results in a representative group and can therefore bias your results. For instance, parents of young children may typically visit a clinic at certain times of the day, people who work full time at other certain times, and older people or those that don't work at still other times. By choosing people who all show up on the same day and time, you are probably picking a certain **subgroup**, and will not hear the opinions of other subgroups.

Validity means that the information you collect accurately describes what is really happening. It's like hitting the bulls-eye on a target.

Reliability means that the measures you are using to collect information remain consistent over time. It's like hitting the same spot on the target (whether on the bulls-eye or not) over and over again.

Obviously – you want both to happen!

Issues of Validity and Reliability

You want the data you collect to be both valid and reliable. Otherwise, the information you get could lead you to the wrong conclusions and seriously diminish the value of the evaluation. There will always be some *error* in your data, but you should take steps to keep such error to an absolute minimum.

Examples of situations that would affect the *validity* of your information:

- The scale that you measure your clients weight on is wrong by 5 lb;
- A question on your survey is frequently misinterpreted to mean something different than what you intended;
- One type of client frequently does not answer the surveys.

An indicator of "frequency of communication between adolescent and parent about HIV" could be measured by one person in terms of number of events per month and another person as a general measure such as "sometimes" or "rarely". What constitutes "communication about HIV" could also be debated (Talked about prevention? Personal risk? Or does just mentioning the subject count?) A better indicator would be "number of times in past 30 days that adolescent has spoken with a parent about any HIV-related topic".

Examples of situations that would affect the *reliability* of your information:

- The scale that you measure your clients weight on tends to 'drift' away from the true value over time, or one of your staff resets the scale every so often;
- You change the wording of several questions on your survey;
- Answers to some questions tend to change depending on current events, who answers the question, how the respondent is feeling, or other external factors.

Issues of validity and reliability need to be considered throughout the evaluation, particularly when you choose your indicators, write your survey or interview guide, recruit people for the evaluation, collect the data, analyze the data, and report the results.

Choosing indicators:

- Be careful that the indicators are clearly worded, so that any two people will understand what they are measuring in the same way.
- Keep indicators consistent over time. Changing an indicator means that you probably can no longer compare information you collected previously with information you collected after the change.
- Use multiple indicators for more complicated objectives, to ensure that you are truly measuring what you want.
- Check the reliability of indicators by asking similar questions in a survey or by asking the same thing at two different time points.

Writing survey or interview guide:

- Pilot test the questions on a handful of people (who are similar to the people you ultimately want to involve) before implementing the survey.
- Put sensitive questions at the end (this includes questions about income, age, and race)
- Be mindful of cultural differences that could affect interpretation of the questions.

Selection bias happens when the group receiving an intervention is different from the group who does not receive the intervention in some way that also affects how their outcomes. Say for example that you choose to offer a new group exercise program to clients at Clinic A, and then compare their outcomes to clients at Clinic B who were not offered the program. You find that the program doesn't work – the clients at Clinic A didn't generally use the program. But perhaps the clients at Clinic A were wealthier than those at Clinic B. They had more options for exercise programs at gyms, and so didn't need a free program. Poorer clients at Clinic B may have responded differently to the intervention. Selection bias partially explains why the program appeared not to work in this case.

Recruiting participants:

- Be wary of *selection bias*. Select people at random whenever possible for the evaluation, and try to ensure that the group of people receiving the program intervention are as similar as possible to the people not receiving the intervention if you intend to make comparisons.
- Be mindful of what your control group will be. A control group is necessary to show that it was the program, and not some external event (change in economic, political or social factors in the population, a new advertising campaign, etc) that caused any changes.
- Try to limit drop-out. People leaving the evaluation before it is complete can cause the same problems as selection bias, above. The people who leave (and

therefore don't provide as much information as those that stay) may be different than those that stay in some way that also affects their outcomes.

Be careful you're your interviewers do not change their style over time. You may need to have 'refresher trainings' to make sure this doesn't happen.

Interviewers may learn how to probe for more information as they get used to the survey or interview, which would lead to different answers over time. Or they might get used to the questionnaire and become sloppy – assuming that people will answer in a certain way because so many have.

You don't want to finish the evaluation and be left to wonder whether the increase in a certain kind of answer was really due to changes brought about by the program – or by changes in how the interviewer asked the question over time!

Collect the data:

- If using a pre-post test design, consider first whether the pretest will influence later responses. For example, if you give clients a pre-test before an educational seminar, they may score better on the post-test simply because they remember the pretest (and not because of your intervention)
- Keep your measurements the same throughout the evaluation. Simply replacing a blood pressure cuff, for example, could suddenly cause all of your clients to have vastly improved blood pressures (when in reality it's just a change in the measurement instrument, and not their real blood pressures)
- Carefully train interviewers and ensure they have the same style. You want differences in your information to be due to real differences in the population, not the way your interviewers ask questions.

Analyze and report the data:

- Keep careful track of how you collect the data so that you can include this information in your analysis and reporting. It is very easy to 'skew' information, and you want to be sure you can justify your methods if any external parties suspect that this has happened.

Chapter 3 checklist—Obtain Data

- ❏ Ethics and confidentiality considered
- ❏ Informed consent written and reviewed
- ❏ Qualitative or quantitative data collection methods chosen
- ❏ Data collection questions pilot tested
- ❏ Sampling method selected
- ❏ Data collected from participants
- ❏ Issues of validity and reliability considered

Chapter 4
Organize & Analyze Data

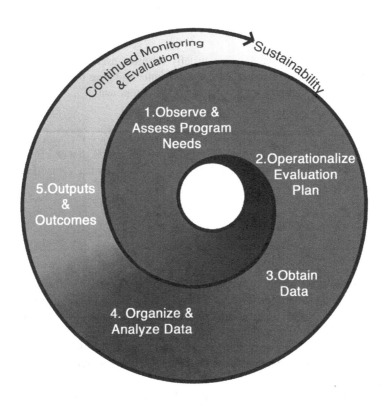

Contents

Introduction to Data Analysis

In Chapter 3 we covered several useful and easy to implement methods for data collection and database creation. This chapter covers the next step in the evaluation process: organizing and analyzing the data that your project has collected. The process of data analysis is used to describe, summarize, and compare data using statistical techniques in a systematic manner. We will only cover basic data analysis techniques in this chapter; for more complex analyses please consult the references at the back of this book.

There are three basic steps in data analysis:

Step 1 – Organizing and preparing the data for analysis
Step 2 – Analyzing the data
Step 3 – Interpreting results

Data organizing and analysis also usually requires user-friendly and flexible software that allows one to create a database to enter and save the information collected and that also includes a solid data analysis component.

The CDC Epi Info website offers a full step-by-step guide to using Epi Info, as well as tutorials and discussion boards where you can get your questions answered.

It's a great resource!

Check it out at www.cdc.gov/epiinfo

As mentioned in Chapter 3, we have found that EPI Info, a software program developed by the Centers for Disease Control (CDC) has all these characteristics. Additionally, to facilitate use of this free program the CDC has developed an extensive guide for community health care programs that gives step-by-step instructions for database creation, data analyses, and for exporting results into a report or presentation. For qualitative data analysis, the CDC has also developed a software for text analysis called EZ-Text.

EPI Info and EZ-text can be downloaded free from www.cdc.gov/epiinfo and www.cdc.gov/hiv/software/ez-text.htm, respectively. However, if your project is already successfully using another software package that allows for simple data analysis, we recommend that you continue using your software package.

The results obtained from analyzing the information entered into your database will help you to:

1. Monitor if your project is progressing as planned.
2. Assess the effect of your project's activities on the knowledge, perceptions, behavior and ultimately on the health of the individuals that your project serves.

3. Share results with your client population, stakeholders within your organization as well as those in your community, local government, and funders. Information about how to present results will be covered in more detail in Chapter 5.

Data collection is not easy. Check your data often to make sure it's as good as you can get.

This includes:

- Reviewing surveys or questionnaires to make sure clients are not skipping parts
- Checking answers randomly to ensure clients are correctly understanding the questions
- Having 2 different people enter the data into a database, then comparing the 2 entries to make sure they are the same
- Checking the final database for irregularities (such as a blood pressure listed as 300/80, or an age or 200, etc), and going back to the original surveys, forms, etc to correct problems

---

Organize and Prepare Data for Analysis

This section will review organizing and preparing data for analysis, including assessing the quality and accuracy of the information collected before entering it into a database, entering the information into the database, keeping a record of sources of data (see Worksheet 5, page 155), and cleaning and preparing the data for ease of analysis.

Data quality—Completed data collection tools (surveys, questionnaires, pre-post tests, etc.) must be verified for quality and accuracy on a regular basis before entering the information into the database. Ideally this type of quality assurance will take place on a daily basis. The person(s) responsible need to have a protocol to address and document inconsistencies or incomplete data, as well as the corrective action taken. The following "decision making tree" (Fig. 4.1) will help you make decisions to assess the quality of the information in your database.

Data entry—If your budget and software program allows, data should be entered twice and then compared to ensure data quality. This is easy to accomplish if using the EPI Info software. The software lets you compare both entries, and highlights entries that were not the same between the two. You can then go back to the original data to figure out the correct answer.

If your program can only afford single data entry, then another protocol for ensuring data quality will need to be developed. For example, the person(s) responsible for supervising data entry could review the information entered into the database against the actual hard copy for every fifth or tenth (or whatever makes sense)

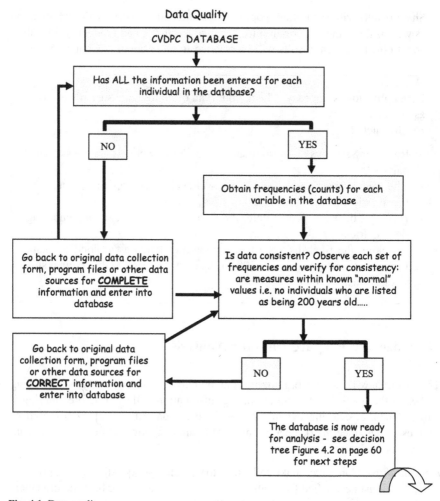

Fig. 4.1 Data quality

hard copy. This would not catch all the mistakes made, however, so the double-entry system is really the best to use whenever possible.

You'd be surprised how many mistakes are made when data are entered into a database, no matter how careful your data entry people are being!

Every mistake that is not caught decreases the quality of the data that you spent all that time and effort collecting!

Avoid this problem by planning on having 2 different people enter the data and using a program like Epi Info to catch places where they don't match. It's much less likely that 2 people will make the same mistake! You can catch most errors this way.

The creation of a **codebook** is also important to describe the information (variables) in the database, and their source (see example of a codebook under Appendix 1, pp. 141).

Preparing Data for Analysis

After making sure that the database is complete and valid, some of the information will need to be organized or transformed into different variables to facilitate the analysis process. For example, if you have collected the age of individual's in your database, it may be difficult to interpret the results when using the raw data on age in relation to an outcome of interest (for example, blood pressure). However, if you create a new variable that could be called "age group" to group the age information into four categories, it would be easier to assess if blood pressure is higher for some age groups than for others.

Example of new variable "age group"

Age group	Number (count of women in each age group)
<30	20
30–40	40
40–50	35
>50	25
All ages	**120**

Whenever you find **missing values** in the database, and if after checking the data collection tool there is no information for that specific value, a point "." should be entered in the empty space to indicate that this value is missing.

Analyze Data

The choice of analysis method depends of the type of evaluation conducted. The following decision making tree will help you to identify the best type of analysis for the information collected (Fig. 4.2).

Analysis of **qualitative data** will not be covered in this section, however, the CDC's EZ-text has solid and simple to follow guidelines for this type of analysis. If you would like a more in-depth understanding of qualitative methodologies, Russell Bernard (1995) provides extensive discussions and examples in his book Research Methods in Anthropology: Qualitative and Quantitative Approaches.

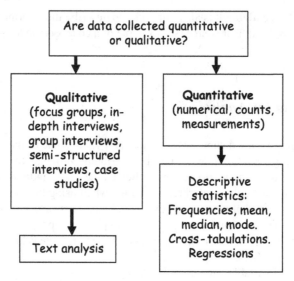

Fig. 4.2 Type of data analysis

Quantitative Data Analysis

Descriptive statistics describe patterns and general trends in a data set. Descriptive statistics are summary measures of what the data shows and can be presented through simple graphs or figures.

> A "frequency" is just a count of events in a given time frame.
> For example, if you report "Our clinic sees 30 patients per month" that's a frequency.
> Frequencies of your variables will be things like:
> 20 females
> 10 males
> 20 with diabetes
> 5 with hypertension
> 5 with neither
> etc.

1. Frequencies

show how data are distributed, giving how many records have each value of a selected variable. A separate frequency table should be created for each variable. An example of a frequency could be the count of clients participating in a program intervention that are female, or the count of age groups shown in the previous example.

2. Mean

The average result of a test, survey, or experiment. In statistics, the mean is the same as the average. To calculate the mean, you add up all the numbers then divide by how many numbers there are (it is the *sum* divided by the *count*).

Although the mean is the most commonly used the median or mode is better.

For example if you tested 10 clients on a knowledge quiz scored from 0–100, and 9 people score above 90 but 1 person scores a 2, the mean will be around 85. That 1 person really throws off the final statistic!

The median would be around 95, however, and in this case is a better description of how most people did.

The mode would answer the question, "what was the most common score?" which could also be very useful.

Example:

Seven people take a test in which 10 points are possible. Their scores are: 2, 3, 5, 8, 8, 9, and 10.

The mean is the sum of the scores (45) divided by the number of people (7). The mean is 6.43.

3. Median

Is a measure of central location where half of the measures are below and the other half are above it.

Example :

Seven people take a test in which 10 points are possible. Their scores are: 2, 3, 5, 8, 8, 9, and 10.

Put the scores in order and a score of 8 is the middle value, therefore the median is 8.

Note the difference in the values between the mean and median. The mean or average can be influenced by extreme or outlying values at either end of the scale but the median is not.

If the number of values is even, there isn't a middle value, so you take the mean of the two middle numbers.

Example: {2, 4, 6, 8, 10, 12}

The two middle numbers are 6 & 8

So the Median = (6 + 8) / 2 = 7

4. Mode

Is the most common result (the most frequent value) of a test, survey, or experiment.

Example :

Seven people take a test in which 10 points are possible. Their scores are: 4, 7, 7, 7, 9, 10, and 10.

Looking at these scores, you can see that 7 is the most common score on the test because three people received a score of 7. The modal score of the test is "7."

5. Proportions or percentage

A proportion, sometimes called relative frequency, is simply the number of times the observation occurs in the data, divided by the total number of responses.

> When reporting percentages, you should also always report *how many* observations there were.
>
> It makes a difference to know that a report like "50% of women seen by the clinic this month had to 50% of 500 women (250 women with diabetes!) or 50% of 2 women (only 1 woman with diabetes).

Example: Proportion of females by age category

Age group	Number (count of women in each age group)	Percent
<30	20	**17**
30–40	40	**33**
40–50	35	**29**
>50	25	**21**
All ages	120	100

6. Cumulative percentage

The cumulative percentage for a given score or data value corresponds to the percent of people who responded with that score or less than that score. You just add the percentage from each group to all of the percentages for groups under it.

Example: Proportion of females by age category

Age	# of women in each age group	Percent	Cumulative percentage
<30	20	17	**17**
30–40	40	33	50
40–50	35	29	79
>50	25	21	100
All ages	120	100	100

Cross-Tabulations Mock Tables

We recommend that you and other staff involved in designing the evaluation plan brainstorm and create "mock tables" as soon as you have finalized your conceptual framework. At the design stage, mock tables will help you decide what type of outcomes are the most important to your program. The tables will stay empty until data have been collected and entered into a database.

The following example of a mock table was created by using the project's conceptual framework to decide which of the program activities would be used as key indicators to track their progress over time.

Percent of clients participating in the CVD Program by type of activity and sex

Type of activity	Sex		Both sexes (n=) %
	Males (n=)%	Females (n=) %	
Education			
Home visits			
Referrals			
Peer training			
Peer educator Community intervention			

With this type of cross-tabulation we could estimate the Chi-Square which is a test of statistical significance that helps us determine how likely it is that an observed association between an exposure and an outcome could have occurred due to chance alone. The Chi-Square Test is a good choice when the expected values for each cell in a two-by-two table are at least five. In some programs such as EPI Info and even Excel software the Chi-Square statistic can be produced.

If you have a program that will calculate the chi-square value for you, it's a helpful number to get and is easy to interpret.

If you found that 40% of women in your clinic attended all sessions, and 8% of men did – this could mean women are better at attending, or it could be that both groups are the same and it was just by hance that you founda difference.

A chi-square result of less than .05 would support the idea that the groups are really different. A score of .05 means that there is only a 5% chance that the groups are really the same, and a 95% chance that the difference is real and women *are* better at attending!

Interpreting the Results

Inferential Statistics

Inferential statistics test hypotheses about differences or relationships in populations on the basis of measurements made on samples. Inferential statistics can help us decide if a difference or relationship can be considered real or is just due to a chance fluctuation.

1. Population and Sample

The entire collection of individuals or measurements about which information is desired is the **population**.

A subset of the population selected for study is the **sample**.

A random sample of size n from a population is a subset of n of the elements from that population where the subset is chosen in such a way that every possible subset of size n has the same chance of being selected as any other.

The goal of inferential statistics is to use sample statistics to make inference about population parameters

---

2. Parameters and Statistics

To find out information about a population, we can do two things:

CENSUS: Look at every object or individual in the population. This takes a lot of time and money.

STATISTICAL INFERENCE: We sample the population (in a manner to ensure that the sample represents the population). We then take measurements on our sample and *infer* (or generalize) back to the population.

Example:

We may want to know the average height of all adults (over 18 years old) in the US. Our population is then all adults over 18 years of age. If we were to census, we would measure every adult and then compute the average. By using statistics, we can take a random sample of adults over 18 years of age, measure their height, and then infer that the average height of the total population is "close to" the average height of our sample.

3. Probability

Example: roll a die, flip a coin, or draw a card from a deck

4. Significance

With what probability the results of research were due to chance.

Significant Difference

Example:

An educational intervention to prevent CVD had one group of participants (Group A) receiving additional educational sessions on increasing physical activity and improving nutritional intake to decrease hypertension, in addition to the standard medical assessment and recommendations. The other group (Group B) only received the standard medical assessment and recommendations. After 2 years in the program participants in Group A had lower blood pressure measures than those in Group B. The study reports a significance of $p < .01$ for the results.

This means that clients enrolled in the enhanced educational sessions had lower blood pressure, there is less than 1 in 100 chance that the results are due to some random factor (such as Group A having smarter participants than Group B).

Note that generally, *p*-values need to be fairly low (.01 and .05 are common) in order for a study to make any strong claims based on the results.

5. Hypotheses

The competing hypotheses are called the **null hypothesis** and the **alternative hypothesis**. Usually, the null hypothesis is that something is not present, that a treatment has no effect, or that there is no difference between two parameters. The alternative hypothesis is that some effect is present, that a treatment has an effect, or that two parameters differ. The main requirement of the null hypothesis is that assuming the null hypothesis is true should make it possible to compute the probability that the test rejects the null hypothesis by chance or the significance level of the test. (When in doubt, choose the simpler of the hypotheses to be the null hypothesis—usually that will lead to easier computations.)

6. *P-value.*

The way in which significance is reported statistically (i.e. $p < .05$ means that there is at least a 5% chance that the results of a study are due to random chance.)
It is conventional in statistics to reject the null hypothesis at the 5% level. The 0.05 level is simply a convenient cutoff value adopted by convention. Values close to 0.05 provide moderate evidence against the null hypothesis, while values less than 0.01 provide considerable evidence against the null hypothesis. However, for programmatic purposes, $p < 1.0$ are sometimes used.

Summary

Evaluation activities, ideally, should be carried out as an integral part of program design to establish the specific needs of the target population. However, in the real world, awareness of the need for evaluation often comes when the program has been ongoing for months and sometimes even for years and only as the result of the need to report progress to the program's funding agencies.

Measuring progress requires having information on the quality of existing services, as well as on the status (health and psychosocial) of the population served right before the implementation of the program's activities, also known as baseline measures, against which subsequent measures can. In Chapter 1, we learned that here are three major types of program evaluation, formative, process (monitoring), and outcome. Each one of these forms of evaluation is ideally suited to assess a program's need, progress or effect on the target population according to the level of program implementation.

Formative Evaluation provides information to help identify the type of program activities that are needed by the target population, and to assess if the planned activities will meet the specific needs of the target population (Fig. 4.3). Formative evaluation results can also serve as the baseline information against which progress can be subsequently measured during the life of the program. Formative evaluation information can be collected and analyzed by using either qualitative or quantitative methods.

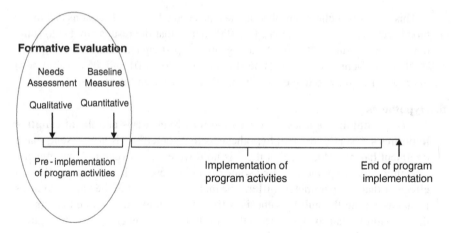

Fig. 4.3 Formative evaluation of a community health care program

Process Evaluation, also known as **monitoring**, uses routinely collected data to assess if the program activities are being implemented as planned, and if they are reaching the target population and not exceeding the allocated budget (Fig. 4.4). Some examples of process evaluation measures include the following: how many program participants received each type of service; how often did they receive the services, and how well were the services provided (measures of quality). Examples of types of data sources include among others: clinic intake records, logs of educational activities, laboratory results, logs with # of ART provided, client satisfaction surveys.

The quality of data thus collected must be assessed on a regular basis and in-house staff training must be conducted regarding the importance of accurate data collection and data recording whether in paper or in electronic format. Data analysis will also be conducted on an ongoing basis.

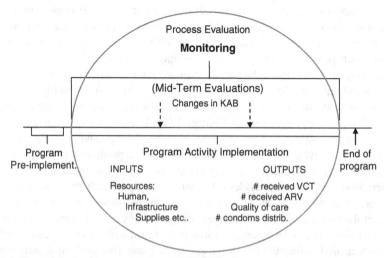

Fig. 4.4 Community health care program (HIV/AIDS)—Process evaluation—Monitoring

Community Health Care Program (HIV/AIDS)—Outcome Evaluation

Outcome Evaluation is used to assess if the program achieved its objectives. Outcome evaluation also asses the effect of the programs activities on the participant's psychosocial, behavioral and ultimately health related outcomes (Fig. 4.5). Cost-benefits analysis is another type of evaluation outcome that can be measured at the end of the program implementation.

Data used for evaluating a program's outcome can be obtained from the program's routinely collected information or, if funding is available, the information can be collected at the end of the program implementation and usually requires the use of a special survey form. Data analysis can be simple (two by two tables with measures of association such as Chi-Square, or complex with the aid of an outside evaluator).

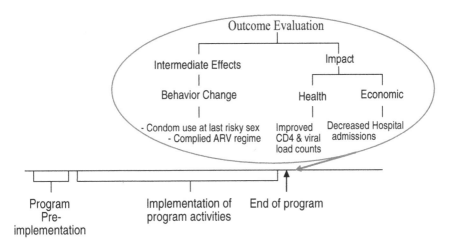

Fig. 4.5 Outcome evaluation

If the program implemented involved a mass media campaign, a survey of a representative sample of the community served (household survey) will be necessary to assess effectiveness of the campaign. Data analysis can be as complex as the sampling methodology and type of data collected and might necessitate an outside evaluator with advance statistical skills.

Community health care organizations vary in available infrastructure, level of funding and in-house capacity in evaluation. However, it has been our experience that most community health care programs are able to design and implement an evaluation plan to help them collect, organize, analyze and disseminate good quality data that provides evidence of the effect of their efforts to improve or maintain the health of the population served. Chapter 5 will cover effective methods for dissemination of your evaluation results.

Chapter 4 checklist—Organize and Analyze Data

❑ Supervision of data quality integrated into evaluation Procedures
❑ Timeline and roles and responsibilities for data management Agreed
❑ Analysis plan reviewed and finalized
❑ Database clean and ready for analysis
❑ Descriptive analysis completed
❑ Outcome analysis completed
❑ Plan for dissemination of evaluation results implemented

Chapter 5
Outputs & Outcomes

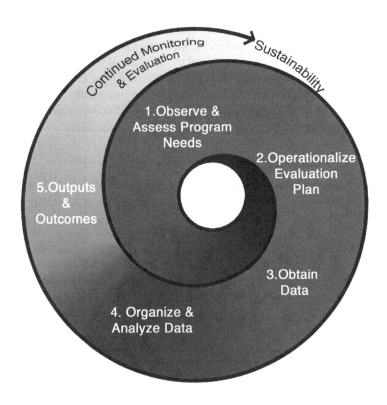

Contents

Outputs & Outcomes

Evaluations are only worthwhile if the results are actually used and reported. This does not have to be a step that happens only at the end of an evaluation, you should consider routinely summarizing and reporting on your outputs and outcomes during the evaluation as well.

Potential Audiences for Results

When you first started planning your evaluation, you and your evaluation team had to decide who the potential audiences would be for your evaluation results. The questions you asked, the information you collected, and even the way you analyzed the results were based on the needs of these audiences. Reporting the outputs and outcomes is no different—the way you do it should be based on the needs of your stakeholders.

Revisit the checklist of stakeholders you identified during the evaluation planning. All of those stakeholders are also audiences for your results. You will likely need to report your progress and results in a variety of different formats to meet the different stakeholder needs.

For this Stakeholder:	Consider as one option:
Your program staff	Presentations at meetings. Keep it simple, with lots of visuals. A short written summary could accompany the presentation.
Board of directors	Quarterly report. Keep it simple and include lots of visual graphs & diagrams
Community members	Newsletter or presentations. Keep it simple, with mainly visuals and pictures.
Policy makers	Written report or press release. Keep it simple, include charts & diagrams.

Note that for every stakeholder mentioned, and for every one not mentioned—the key is to keep it simple and have visual images included. If you can say it with a picture or graph, then do so.

Creating Graphs & Tables

There are many different ways to create visual images of your data, depending on the type of data you have and what you want to say with it. Below are a few of the more common ways, all of which can be created using most word processing, spreadsheet, or statistical computer programs.

Tables are useful for when you have a lot of data that you want to show that would be confusing if written out. They can be used for either quantitative or qualitative data. An example of a good table would be:

Southern primary healthcare clinics CDPC[a] program systolic and diastolic blood pressure at baseline and at 1-year follow-up by client's sex

	Males		Females	
	Baseline (n=27) %	Follow-up (n=27) %	Baseline (n=48) %	Follow-up (n=47) %
Systolic				
Normal (90–129)	33	50	33	47
Med/high (130–140)	52	46	50	38
High (150–200)	15	4	17	15
Diastolic				
Normal (50–89)	67	96	76	87
Med/high (90–99)	33	4	14	13
High (100–150)	0	0	10	0

[a] Cardiovascular disease prevention & control.

What makes it a 'good' table?

- Numbers are rounded to whole numbers (you shouldn't ever need to report more than 1 decimal place unless you're talking about money—and even then it clutters up the table and does not add much value).
- There's enough 'white space' so the table doesn't appear crowded or cluttered.
- The layout makes it easy to follow, with groups of information separated by lines, indents or spaces so they are clearly distinguishable.
- Someone reading the table could understand what it's about without having to read any outside text at all.

Pie Charts are great for showing percentages. An example of a good pie chart would be:

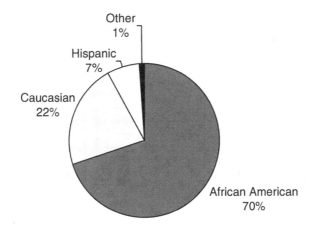

Racial demographics of counties served by Southern Primary HealthCare Clinics, 2005

What makes it a 'good' pie chart?

- All the 'pieces' add up to 100%
- Different patterns clearly separate the pieces, making it easier to read.
- A reader can understand what the data says without having to read any text outside of the chart.

Bar graphs are great for comparing numbers or percentages. Examples of good bar graphs would be:

Percent change in CVD risk for intervention and comparison groups at baseline and follow-up

Why are they 'good' bar graphs?

- A reader can understand them without having to read any text outside of the graphs.

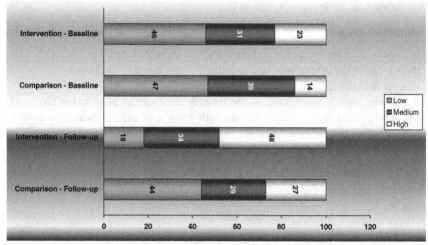

*CDPC – cardiovascular disease prevention & Control program, Southern Primary HealthCare clinics

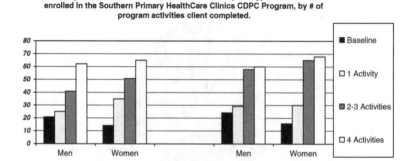

Knowledge and attitudes at baseline and at follow-up for hypertensive clients enrolled in the Southern Primary HealthCare Clinics CDPC Program, by # of program activities client completed.

- Labels and spacing make them easy to read, and easy to see the comparisons between groups.

Line graphs are useful when showing how much something has changed over time, or when comparing changes in different groups over time. An example of a good line graph would be:

Average blood pressure level for clients enrolled in the Southern Primary HealthCare Clinics CDPC Program, at baseline and follow-ups, by sex

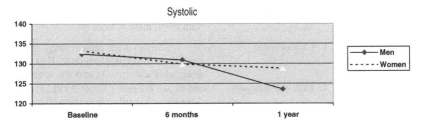

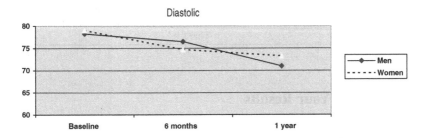

What makes it a 'good' line graph?

- There aren't too many lines (not cluttered or confusing)
- Labeling makes it easy for a reader to understand what the data says without having to read a description in the text.

Tables and charts can also be used for qualitative data. Consider the following examples:

Top three most commonly cited barriers to routine exercise by women in open-ended survey question, by age group

Respondents	Top three most common themes	Examples of comments
Women >50 years	1. Lack of companionship	'Sara and me used to walk together a lot, but then she moved away. I'm not interested in walking alone.'
	2. Concerns about injury	'I fell on the sidewalk 3 months ago and it took 10 minutes for someone to come by and help me. I'm not going to risk that again.'
	3. Concerns about safety	'Where am I going to go exercise? I don't have a car to get to any park, and my neighborhood ain't safe to walk around in.'

(continued)

Table (continued)

Respondents	Top three most common themes	Examples of comments
Women 30–50 years	1. Lack of Time	'I don't have any time for exercise. I think I get enough running between 2 jobs and my kids!'
	2. Concerns about safety	'I tell my teenage son to stay in after school and play video games inside, and I stay in, too. It's not safe to be out and about in our neighborhood.'
	3. Lack of companionship	'It's kind a boring to go exercise on your own. I probably would if I had someone to go with me to make it more fun.'
Women <30 years	1. Lack of Time	'As it is I hardly ever get enough sleep, and can't seem to get anything done. How am I going to fit a daily walk into that schedule?'
	2. Family obligations	'I used to jog, but now I've got 3 kids, 1, 3 and 5, and it's too hard to drag them all along. And I don't have anyone to leave them with so I could go jog alone.'
	3. Concerns about safety	'It's not safe where I live to walk around. I walk to the bus station in the morning, and I have a friend drive me home if I get off after dark. That's it.'

Ways to Report Your Results

Written Reports

Regardless of who else you will be sharing evaluation results with, you should prepare a written report of the evaluation for your own use. Some tips about writing an evaluation report:

- Keep it simple. It is easy to get bogged down in mounds of information, but you don't want *all* of that in your report. Decide what the main findings are from the evaluation, and focus on them.
- If you can show your data in a table or graph format, then do so. Graphics made the report look more appealing to the reader than just straight text for pages and pages. Don't explain the graphics in the text, just reference them. Let the tables and graphs speak for themselves through good labeling.
- Use bullet points, lists or tables whenever possible. They're easier to read than large paragraphs of text.
- Do not assume the reader knows anything about your project or the evaluation. Explain everything (briefly), and keep the language simple. The rule of thumb is to write at an eighth-grade level. Even if your audience is a group of professionals, everyone appreciates having an easy-to-read document.

> Protect the confidentiality of your participants. Be sure that nothing in any part of the report can be used to identify individual participants.

- Be honest in your reporting, and do not leave out or downplay 'negative' results. All evaluations result in both positive and negative findings, and it is important that you represent both fairly. Positive findings make you happy, but negative findings tell you how to improve, so they're very important! Be careful also in your tables and graphs that you don't format them in a way that misrepresents the data.

The basic format of an evaluation report is:

1. Title page
2. Executive Summary
3. Purpose (why you did the evaluation)
4. Description of Project
5. Description of evaluation methods used
6. Results
7. Discussion
8. Recommendations and future actions
9. Appendices

Executive Summary

The executive summary is a concise review of the entire report. It is often the only part that people read, so make sure it goes over all the key points, important findings, and final recommendations.

> The executive summary may be the only thing some people ever read from your report. Make sure it contains all the information that you consider important, and that is kept brief and interesting!

- Keep it short—one page is best, more than four is too many.
- Put contact information at the end (project name, address, phone, and date), as often the executive summary is taken away from a full report and distributed by itself.
- Write it last, after you have completed the rest of the report *and* gotten feedback on it from other project staff or stakeholders.

Purpose

Give a background of the evaluation project so readers know what to expect in the report. Why did you conduct an evaluation? What questions were you hoping to answer?

Background

Give a background of your project. How is your project organized, what services does it provide, and what is its history?

- Be fairly brief, but include enough information that the reader can understand what the evaluation results mean, and why you made the final recommendations that you did.
- Details you may want to include might be:
  - where the project works (in a clinic, in schools, at community gathering places, etc);
  - what kind of resources does your program have (offices, clinics, number of staff, organizational structure, etc)
  - who the project serves (types and numbers of people, organizations, or events that receive program services);
  - other groups involved (community organizations, etc. that collaborate on the program activities);
  - program history (why were the specific interventions chosen, when were they first offered, and how and why has the program changed from the original vision);
  - etc.

> The background section is only to give the reader an idea of what your program is and how it fits into the community. It is NOT a place to describe at length the whole history of your program. Focus on the important details – the ones that will help the reader understand what your program is all about.

Methods

This section is where you detail what you did during the evaluation. Describe the data collection methods you used, and include all important details.

- Do not be afraid to make this section longer. In this case, it is more important to have all the details than to be brief.
- Include information on:
  - how you choose the participants in your evaluation,
  - whether you excluded anyone,
  - whether any information was gathered but not used,
  - what the response rates were,
  - how the data collection tools were created (did you develop your own or borrow one?),
  - how you performed data analysis,
  - how you entered or stored the information you collected, etc.

- The rule of thumb for this section is to be detailed enough that another person could come along and repeat your evaluation just by reading your methods section. Think of it as a 'how-to' guide for your evaluation.

Results

Summarize the results obtained from your evaluation.

- Use table, charts or graphs whenever possible. Mention the key points of each graphic in the text of the report, but let the graphic do most of the 'talking' by itself (in other words, don't write out everything that the graph shows, just mention the most important thing about it).

Don't go overboard in reporting results. Just include those results that you deem to be the most critical. Summarize whenever possible. You can always add an appendix to your report with all the rest of your results.

- Organize the results in a logical fashion. This doesn't have to be in the order that they were obtained.
- Do not talk about what the results mean, whether they were 'positive' or 'negative', whether they were a surprise, etc. This section just lists the facts. You will discuss what you think about the facts, and what they might mean, in the next section of the report.

Talk about possible explanations for the results other than the one you have given. For instance, perhaps it wasn't your program that decreased smoking, maybe it was just a trend that is happening everywhere and would have happened even without your program. Or maybe a tax increase on the price of cigarettes caused the change. Once you have listed the strongest alternative explanations, discuss why you believe your explanation is correct. Back this up with outside information and references whenever possible.

Discussion

In this section go back to the main results and describe what they might mean.

- This is where you take all the facts and pull them together into a story. Using the detective analogy again, if you were a detective, this would be where you would gather all the evidence and report your best guess at what it all means.
- Discuss strengths of your evaluation, and reference other literature, evaluation reports, or information if it helps explain or support your conclusions.

- Make sure to get feedback on this section (as well as other sections), as you may find that other stakeholders reach very different conclusions from the same information.
- Talk about problems with the evaluation, limitations to the information you gathered, and other possible explanations for the findings. For example, if response to the survey was very high among women but very low among men, this might be a limitation, as there may be differences between them and you may not have enough information from men to make a valid conclusion.

Recommendations

From what you presented in the results and discussion, discuss how the evaluation results should be used.

Double and triple-check your final report and all appendices to make sure:

- Spelling and grammar are correct
- Charts, graphs, and tables are well labeled and can be understood without reading the main text
- Formatting is clean and consistent
- There is enough 'white space' to make each page look appealing to the eye
- Contact information is included in the executive summary and at the end of the report
- There is no information anywhere in the report that could identify any of the participants in your evaluation.

- Make sure to be clear about who the recommendation are directed towards, and who should take the action.
- Recommendations may be to change or improve your own project, and may also be to make changes external to your project (such as policy changes, etc).
- Discuss surprises, set-backs, problems, and successes of the evaluation, and also recommend actions for the next evaluation.
- This is another section that it is very important to get feedback on, as there is often disagreement about what actions should be taken (and by whom) based on the evaluation results.

Appendices

Attach useful documents or information. Example of things you should consider attaching:

- Copies of the surveys, questionnaires, or interviewer guides that you used for data collection
- The consent form that you used for participants

- Articles or other short reports that help explain your evaluation report
- Detailed results that were too long for the actual report, such as the full results from group interviews, one-on-one interviews, survey results, etc.

Presentations

Presentations are excellent ways to present your findings to different groups. You can do a presentation for your own project staff, at professional meetings or conferences, at community gatherings, or other forums.

The key to a good presentation is to make it into an interesting, but brief, story. Start with an introduction of the project and the evaluation, briefly mention how the evaluation was conducted, and give a summary of results. Close it up with a discussion of what it all means, and state your recommendations.

Keep your presentation to just the key points, and let the audience fill in the rest by asking questions. Make heavy use of visual aids. You can use a computer-generated display, an overhead projector, a flip chart, or posters, but have some sort of visuals. Make sure the visuals are simple, too. Don't crowd your visuals with text or too much information—just hit the key points.

Newsletters

Newsletters are great to keep stakeholders updated about the progress of your evaluation, and to provide a continual forum for their feedback (by you including contact information and a request for feedback in each newsletter).

Keep the information brief and clear, and use pictures, quotes or other interesting visuals as additions to the text. Develop a standard timeline for your newsletters, so stakeholders know when they can expect the next update and aren't left guessing.

Press Releases

Press releases are given to the media for reporting. They must be kept brief (one–four single sided pages at most), and should be very clear (avoid jargon!). State the key point in the first few lines, and then fill in the important details. Make sure to include contact information in case they want to follow-up or get more information. Send the release to several places (newspapers, journals, radio stations, etc) at the same time. Follow up to make sure it was received and to see if they need more information.

> Press releases must be very short and very interesting in order to gain attention. Focus on the community impact of your program to heighten the appeal.

Other Formats

Website

If your project has a website, post the evaluation results on one of the website pages. You can actually post a lot of detailed information, more so than you would put in a written report or presentation (being careful again to protect the confidentiality of participants), and then reference the website in the report or presentation as being an extra source of information.

Fact Sheet

Fact sheets are best when they are a single page (can be a double-sided page) with a bullet-pointed list of major evaluation findings. Make them pleasing to look at (use some color, add a photo, and make generous use of 'white space'), and you can hand them out to clients, politicians, community members, or other stakeholders.

Video

A short video presentation can be a great way to present your evaluation findings. Consider it a mix between a regular presentation and a press release. You want to keep it brief and to the point, and develop it as much as possible into a 'story' to make it somewhat interesting. Simply recording a standard presentation that you give, and then filling it in with extra pictures, graphics, or dialogue, can be an easy way to do this.

Interpreting & Using Results

You've made it all the way through designing, implementing, analyzing, and reporting on an evaluation. Don't call it quits here, though! To make the whole thing worthwhile, you have to make sure the results of your hard work get *used*.
Evaluation results are of great value both to your own organization and to others outside of your organization. Following is a brief list of some ways that your results should be put to good use.

Improve Your Program

Evaluation results highlight the strengths of your program, and also call attention to some weaknesses. Staff can use the results to build on your strengths and work on improving weak spots.

Train Your Staff

Use the evaluation results to point out aspects of the program that work really well, or that don't work very well at all. Use both to train staff, so they know what to do (or what not to do).

Plan for the Future

Will you continue your program exactly as is, or did the evaluation reveal potential new directions for the program results to consider changes in your program.

Promote Your Program

Use your evaluation results to enhance your public image and make others aware of the benefits of your program. Results can also be used to inform other organizations of your work and to form partnerships with those organizations.

Gain Funding

Funders want to know what is done with their investment, and what sort of positive changes were achieved. Including evaluation results, as well as plans for future evaluations, can really help boost your program's chances of gaining more funds.

Influence Policy

Use your evaluation results to convince policy makers of changes that need to be made for the community. Policy makers respond well to charts and numbers, and including a few comments from participants can add a personal touch and really drive the message home.

Planning for Continued Evaluation of the Program

Evaluation is not a one-time deal. To ensure the long-term sustainability of your program, monitoring and evaluation activities should be ongoing activities. The good news is, monitoring and evaluation becomes much easier once you have already gone through it once. And once it is clear how evaluation results can help gain additional funding, promote your program, and improve your services, you will want evaluation to be an indispensable part of your activities.

Discuss with your evaluation team how you feel evaluation efforts could best be continued. It is good to decide to continue to meet as a team at regular intervals, and to continue to collect process data. At the routine meetings, the team can decide whether or not it is time to again collect participant data, or whether to begin evaluation for another part of your organization's activities.

For future projects, you should consider including the cost of an outside evaluator into your grant applications. An outside evaluator will free up more of your staff time and will be able to perform more complex forms of evaluation. And since your staff will have performed one evaluation on their own, they will be well prepared to guide an outside evaluator and ensure that the evaluation is done properly.

Monitoring and evaluation, when done well and put to good use, truly can help ensure the long-term sustainability of your program. We hope this guide has helped you get started, and we wish you and your project many years of positive, productive evaluations!

Chapter 5 checklist—Outputs and Outcomes

- ❑ Audiences for evaluation results identified
- ❑ Decision of format to present results
- ❑ Creation of tables or graphs of data
- ❑ Evaluation report drafted
- ❑ Presentation & dissemination of results
- ❑ Interpretation and use of results to improve program
- ❑ Plan for continuing evaluation efforts

Bibliography

Adamchak, S., Bond, K., MacLaren, L., Magnani, R., Nelson, K., & Seltzer, J. "A Guide to Monitoring and Evaluating Adolescent Reproductive Health Programs. FOCUS on Young Adults Tool Series 5, June 2000." Washington, DC: FOCUS on Young Adults (2000). http://www.pathfind.org/pf/pubs/focus/guidesandtools/PDF/part%20I.pdf & http://wwwpathfind.org/pf/pubs/focus/guidesandtools/PDF/part%20II.pdf. Accessed 4/4/05.

Bernard, H.R. "Research Methods in Anthropology: Qualitative and Quantitative Approaches." 2nd edition. Walnut Creek, CA: Altamira Press, Sage Publication (1995).

Bond, S., Boyd, S., & Rapp, K. "Taking Stock, A Practical Guide to Evaluating Your Own Programs." Chapel Hill: Horizon Research, Inc. (1997). http://www.horizon-research.com/reports/1997/stock.pdf. Accessed 3/25/05.

CORE Initiative. "Participatory Monitoring and Evaluation of Community- and Faith-Based Programs." Washington, DC: CORE Initiative (2004) http://www.coreinitiative.org/Resources/Publications/PME_manual/

Epi Info™. "Software for Database Creation, Management, Analysis and Presentation." Version 3.3.2. Atlanta, GA: Centers for Disease Control and Prevention (CDC) (2005). Download the software from: http://www.cdc.gov/epiinfo/. Accessed 2/12/07.

EPI INFO™. "Community Health Assessment Tutorial." Version 2.0. Atlanta, GA: Department of Health and Human Services, Centers for Disease Control and Prevention (CDC). (2005).

The tutorial manual can be downloaded from: http://www.cdc.gov/epiinfo/communityhealth.htm. Accessed 2/10/07.

Johnson, A. "Engaging Queenslanders: Evaluating Community Engagement." Brisbane: Queensland Government Department of Communities (2004). http://www.getinvolved.qld.gov.au/share_your_knowledge/resources/documents/pdf/guide_evaluation.pdf. Accessed 4/6/05.

MacDonald, G., Starr, G., Schooley, M., Yee, S.L., Klimowski, K., & Turner, K. "Introduction to Program Evaluation for Comprehensive Tobacco Control Programs". Atlanta, GA: Centers for Disease Control and Prevention (CDC). (2001). http://www.cdc.gov/tobacco/evaluation_manual/evaluation.pdf. Accessed 3/25/05.

MEASURE Evaluation . "Compilation of Evaluation Publications." http://www.cpc.unc.edu/measure/publications/index.php?searchterm=All&page=next&offset=0. Accessed January 2006.

"Program Development and Evaluation." Evaluation publications. University of Wisconsin-Extension (1996). http://www.uwex.edu/ces/pdande/evaluation/evaldocs/html. Accessed 3/24/05. (series of documents)

Rogers, E.M. "Diffussion of Innovations." 5th edition. New York, NY: Free Press (2003).

Rossi, P.H., & Freeman, H.E. "Evaluation. A Systematic Approach." 5th edition. Newbury Park, CA: Sage Publications (1993).

"Toolkit: A User's Guide to Evaluation for National Service Programs." Burlingame: Project Star, Corporation for National Service (2003). http://www.projectstar.org/star/library/toolkit.html. Accessed 3/23/05.

SRI International. "We Did It Ourselves: An Evaluation Guide Book." Sacramento: Sierra Health
    Foundation (2000). (print copy only)
UNAIDS. "Tools for Evaluating HIV Voluntary Counseling and Testing." Best Practice Collection
    00.009E. Geneva, Switzerland (2000). http:/www.unaids.org
Valente, T.W. "Foundations of Program Evaluation: Theories of Practice." Newbury Park, CA:
    Sage Publications (2002).
Valente, T.W. "Network Models of the Diffusion of Innovations." Cresskill, NJ: Hampton Press
    (1995).
Wasserman, S., & Galaskiewicz, J. "Advances in Social Network Analysis: Research in the Social
    and Behavioral Sciences." Newbury Park, CA: Sage Publications (1994).

Literature Review Matrix — Evaluation Handbooks

Code: 0=Not mentioned, 1=Mentioned, little detail, 2=Topic covered, 3=Extensive discussion of topic. L=Link to other source, C=Checklist, R=References, T=Table/chart/picture, W=Worksheet, X=Examples

Reference	Format/design	Target population	Overview/description	Why, how, when & for	Types of eval.	Decision-making tree	Logic models	Objectives/indicators	Stakeholders	Data collection	Software for data	Eval questions	Ethical considerations	Budget/resources	Quantitative analysis	Qualitative analysis	Data quality/standards	Interpretation/action	Reporting results	Outside evaluators	Pitfalls/FAQs/barriers	Other
"A UNICEF Guide for Monitoring and Evaluation: Making a Difference?" UNICEF. http://www.unicef.org/reseval/index.html Accessed April 4, 2005.																						
Johnson, AL (Nov 2004) "Engaging Queenslanders: Evaluating Community Engagement." Queensland Government Department of Communities. http://www.getinvolved.qld.gov.au/share_your_knowledge/resources/documents/pdf/guide_evaluation.pdf Accessed April 6, 2005.	1 - how-to in pdf	Public officials engaged in community involvement projects	2	2	2	0	2 T X	2 X	2	2 X	0	2 X	2	0	1	1	1	2	2	2	0	Case study; summaries at end of each section; glossary; references

Literature Review Matrix — Evaluation Handbooks

Code: 0=Not mentioned, 1=Mentioned, little detail, 2=Topic covered, 3=Extensive discussion of topic.   L=Link to other source, C=Checklist, R=References, T=Table/chart/picture, W=Worksheet, X=Examples

Reference	Format/design	Target population	Overview/description	Why, how, when & for	Types of eval.	Decision-making tree	Logic models	Objectives/indicators	Stakeholders	Data collection	Software for data	Eval questions	Ethical considerations	Budget/resources	Quantitative analysis	Qualitative analysis	Data quality/standards	Interpretation/action	Reporting results	Outside evaluators	Pitfalls/FAQs/barriers	Other
MacDonald et al. (2001) "Introduction to Program Evaluation for Comprehensive Tobacco Control Programs." CDC, Department of Health & Human Services. http://www.cdc.gov/tobacco/evaluation_manual/Evaluation.pdf. Accessed March 25, 2005.	1 - how-to in pdf	State tobacco control managers	2 T	1	2 C R	0	2 T X	2 T X	3 C R X	2 R T	0	1	0	1	1	1	2 C	2 C	2 C L R T	2 C	0	Sample state evaluation reports; table of data sources with contact info; references; glossary
"Toolkit: A User's Guide to Evaluation for National Service Programs." Burlingame: Project Star, Corporation for National Service. http://www.projectstar.og/star/Library/toolkit.html. Accessed March 23, 2005.	1 - how-to in pdf	Americorps volunteers	2	0	0	0	0	3 W X	2	2 W X	2 T	3 W X	1	0	2 T W X	2 W X	0	1	2 C W X	0	0	Training worksheets at end; Nice beginners guide to compiling & counting data for analysis

Reference	Format	Audience																			Notes
Adamchak et al. (June 2000) "A Guide to Monitoring and Evaluating Adolescent Reproductive Health Programs: FOCUS on Young Adults Tool Series 5." Washington, DC: FOCUS on Young ADults. http://www.pathfind.org/pf/pubs/focus/guidesandtools/PDF/part%20I.pdf and /part%20II.pdf. Accessed April 4, 2005.	1 – how-to in pdf	Program managers of reproductive health programs	2	2	2 C	0	3 T W X	2	2 T W	1	2	2	2 W	2 T W X	1	2	0	2	2	2	Full appendices on sample size, sampling and large list of indicators; glossary; reference list & websites
Bond, Boyd & Rapp (1997) "Taking Stock: A Practical Guide to Evaluating Your Own Programs." Chapel Hill. Horizon Research, Inc: http://www.horizon-research.com/reports/1997/stock.pdf. Accessed March 25, 2005.	1 – how-to in pdf	CBOs	1	2 X	2 X	1	2 T X	0	2 X	0	2	0	1	2 T X	2 T X	0	0	1 X	1	0	Glossary; 2 full case-studies that read through sample eval start to finish, 2 full eval-reports & a full grant proposal example
Guijt, I & Woodhill, J (2002) "Managing for Impact in Rural Development: A Guide for Project M&E." IFAD (International Fund for Agricultural Development). http://www.ifad.org/evaluation/guide/index.htm. Accessed April 26, 2005.	1 – how-to in pdf	Those working on rural development programs	3	2 R	0	2 R T X	3 T	2	3 R X	0	0	0	2 T X	2	2	2	3 C T X	2 R	0	2	Glossary, appendix on data collection,
Shaw, AT & Racine, YA (Nov 2004) Evaluation Toolkit for Community Youth Programmers. Offord Centre for Child Studies, McMaster Children's Hospital-McMaster University. http://www.offordcentre.com/rsd/hac/pdf/HAC%20Report%20Final_web.pdf. Accessed April 21, 2005.	1 – how-to in pdf	Community youth programmers	0	2	2	2 T	2 T W	2	2 W X	0	1	2	0	2	2	2	2	1	0	2	Info on protecting data, coding, etc.

Literature Review Matrix — Evaluation Handbooks

Code: 0=Not mentioned, 1=Mentioned, little detail, 2=Topic covered, 3=Extensive discussion of topic.   L=Link to other source, C=Checklist, R=References, T=Table/chart/picture, W=Worksheet, X=Examples

Reference	Format/design	Target population	Overview/description	Why, how, when & for	Types of eval.	Decision-making tree	Logic models	Objectives/indicators	Stakeholders	Data collection	Software for data	Eval questions	Ethical considerations	Budget/resources	Quantitative analysis	Qualitative analysis	Data quality/standards	Interpretation/action	Reporting results	Outside evaluators	Pitfalls/FAQs/barriers	Other
SRI International (2000) "We Did It Ourselves: An Evaluation Guide Book." Sacramento, CA: Sierra Health Foundation	1 - how-to in pdf	CBOs	2	2	1	0	0	2 W	0	2 T X	2 R	2 T	0	2	2 W X	1	2	1	2 T	0	1	Glossary; refs. appendices on sample indicators, sample surveys & coding examples, analysis,
Westat, JF (Jan 2002) "The 2002 User-Friendly Handbook for Project Evaluation" National Science Foundation. http://www.nsf.gov/pubs/2002/nsf02057/nsf02057.pdf. Accessed March 23, 2005.	1 - how-to in pdf	Managers working with NSF — to evaluate NSF educational programs	2	2	2 R T	0	2 T X	2 R W	2 W	3 L R T	1	2	1	1	2 R T	2 R T	2 T	2	2 R T	2	0	Discusses bias in data collection; advantages/disadvantages to many methods; glossary; references
Various authors (1996) "Program Development and Evaluation — Evaluation Publications". University of Wisconsin-Extension. http://www.uwex.edu/ces/pdande/evaluation/evaldocs.html. Accessed March 24, 2005. (series of documents)	1 - how-to in pdf	Extension program directors	0	2 T	0	0	0	2 X	1	2 R T T X	2 R T T X	3 R T X	1	1	3 T X	3 L R T X	2	1	2 R T X	0	0	Overall planning worksheet

Reference	Type	Audience	1	2	3	4	5	6	7	8	9	10	11	12	13	14	15	16	17	18	Notes
Frechtling & Westat, eds. (1997) "User-Friendly Handbook for Mixed Method Evaluations." National Science Foundation, Division of Research, Evaluation & Communication. http://www.ehr.nsf.gov/HER/REC/pubs/NSF97-153/start.htm. Accessed March 28, 2005.	2 - how-to guide in html	Project directors interested in qualitative methods	2 R	2	1	0	0	2 W	2 W	3 R	1	2 W	1	1	3 R T W	1	2	2 T	0	0	Annotated bibliography with descriptions of references
(Oct 2004) "Monitoring and Evaluation Toolkit" RHRC Consortium. http://www.rhrc.org/resources/general_fieldtools/toolkit/index.htm. Accessed April 21, 2005.	2 - how-to guide in html	Program managers																			
McNamara, C. "Basic Guide to Program Evaluation." http://www.mapnp.org/library/evaluatn/fnl_eval.htm. Accessed March 22, 2005.	2 - how-to guide in html	For profits & non-profits	2	2 C	2 L	0	0	1	1 L	2 L	0	0 L	1 X	0	1 L	1	1	1	1	1	List of other resources at end with links; overall 'Checklist for Program Evaluation Planning'
University of Kansas. 'Community Toolbox': Evaluate Initiative tool.' http://ctb.ku.edu/tools/evaluateinitiative/index.jsp. Accessed March 22, 2005.	2 - how-to guide in html	Community based Org's		2 L	1 L	0	1 L W	1 L T	1 L	2 L	1 L	1 L			1 L		2 X	1 L		3	Library of weblinks; examples of 'evaluating initiatives'
W.K. Kellogg Foundation. "Evaluation Toolkit." http://www.wkkf.org/Programming/Extra.aspx?CID=281&ID=2.	2 - how-to guide in html	Kellogg grantees; non-profits	0	2	2 C L R T	0	1 L W	2 L T W	2 W	2 L R W X	0	2 L R X	2 L R X	2 W	2 L R	1	2 X	2	3 C L R	2	Extensive links to textbook chapters, other resources

Literature Review Matrix — Evaluation Handbooks

Code: 0=Not mentioned, 1=Mentioned, little detail, 2=Topic covered, 3=Extensive discussion of topic. L=Link to other source, C=Checklist, R=References, T=Table/chart/picture, W=Worksheet, X=Examples

Reference	Format/design	Target population	Overview/description-	Why, how, when & for	Types of eval.	Decision-making tree	Logic models	Objectives/indicators	Stakeholders	Data collection	Software for data	Eval questions	Ethical considerations	Budget/resources	Quantitative analysis	Qualitative analysis	Data quality/standards	Interpretation/action	Reporting results	Outside evaluators	Pitfalls/FAQs/barriers	Other
CSAP's Prevention Pathways, Online Courses. "Evaluation for the Unevaluated: Program Evaluation 101, 102 & 201." http://pathwayscourses.samhsa.gov. Accessed March 23, 2005.	3 - how-to in online interactive format	People new to evaluation	2	2	2 R T	0	0	1	0	2 L X	0	2 X	2 L X	1	3 L X	0	2 R X	2	2	2	3	Entire training module on statistics (t-tests, correlation, sub-group analysis, etc); quizzes, glossary
South Australian Community Health Research Unit. "Planning and Evaluation Wizard." http://www.sachru.sa.gov.au/pew/howto/navframe.htm. Accessed March 28, 2005.	3 - how-to in online interactive format	Beginners	2	2	2	0	0	2 C R X	0	2 C L X	0	1	3 L R	2 X	0	0	1	1	2 X	2	0	Excel budget worksheet
"Evaluating Health Promotion Programs: Version 3.3 October 21, 2002." University of Toronto, The Health Communication Unit at the Centre for Health Promotion. http://www.thcu.ca/infoandresources/evaluation_resources.htm#tp. Accessed March 24, 2005.	4 - overview in pdf	Health promotion practitioners	2	3 T	2 R T W	1 T	2 W	2 W X	3 W	2 R T W	1	2 C R	2 C	3 R T W X	2 R T	2 R T	2	2	2 C R X	0	0	Very nice list of references.

Citation	Type	Audience																		Notes
Anderson & Abdalla (2000) "A Step-by-Step Guide to Planning and Implementing Evaluation Strategies." George Mason University. http://www.caph.gmu.edu/VA_ABC_StepByStepFall2000.pdf. Accessed April 25, 2005.	4 - overview in pdf	Program manager or coordinator	1 W	1	0	0	1 W	1 W	0	1 W	0	1 W	1	1 W	0	1 W	1 W	0	0	
Burt et al. (1997) "Evaluation Guidebook: For Projects Funded by S.T.O.P. Formula Grandts Under the Violence Against Women Act." Washington, DC: Urban Institute. http://www.urban.org/UploadedPDF/guidebook.pdf. Accessed April 20, 2005.	4 - overview in pdf	Those working on s.t.o.p. grants for violence against women	2	2 T	2 T W	1 W	0	1 W	2 X	1 W	0	2	2	2	0	2	0	2	2	Chapters on objectives and evaluation details for different types of programs; list of different measurement scales
SAMHSA (2002) "Achieving Outcomes: A Practitioner's Guide to Effective Prevention." US Department of Health and Human Services. http://modelprograms.samhsa.gov/pdfs/AchievingOutcomes.pdf. Accessed April 25, 2005.	4 - overview in pdf	Program manager	2 T	2	3	2	2	2	0	2	1	1	2	2	0	2	0	2	0	Good overview of cultural competency in Chapter 4
"Why Evaluate?" Americans for the Arts, Youth Arts. http://www.americansforthearts.org/youtharts/pdf/evaluation.pdf. Accessed March 24, 2005.	4 - overview pdf	Program managers of at-risk youth arts programs	2	2	2	1	1	2	0	2 R	0	2 X	1 X	1	0	1 X	2	0	1	List of other resources
(1998) "An Educator's Guide to Evaluating the Use of Technology in Schools and Classrooms." US Department of Education. http://www.ed.gov/pubs/EdTechGuide/index.html. Accessed March 24, 2005.	4 - overview pdf	Educators who want to evaluate technology in the classroom	2 T	2 W X	0	0	2 T W X	0	2 T W X	0	2 W X	0	2 T W X	2 T W X	0	2 T W X	2 T W X	0	0	Examples of technology surveys

Literature Review Matrix — Evaluation Handbooks

Code: 0=Not mentioned, 1=Mentioned, little detail, 2=Topic covered, 3=Extensive discussion of topic.   L=Link to other source, C=Checklist, R=References, T=Table/chart/picture, W=Worksheet, X=Examples

Reference	Format/ design	Target population	Overview/ description	Why, how, when & for	Types of eval.	Decision-making tree	Logic models	Objectives/indicators	Stakeholders	Data collection	Software for data	Eval questions	Ethical considerations	Budget/resources	Quantitative analysis	Qualitative analysis	Data quality/standards	Interpretation/action	Reporting results	Outside evaluators	Pitfalls/FAQs/barriers	Other
Atkinson & Ashton (2002) "Planning for Results: The Safe and Drug-Free Schools and Communities Program Planning and Evaluation Handbook." Department of Education, Viginia. http://www.safeanddrugfreeva.org/planningforresults.pdf. Accessed March 25, 2005.	4 - overview pdf	People implementing safe & drug-free schools & communities programs	1	2	2 L R T	0	1 X	2 W X	1	2 T	1	0	0	1	2 X	1	2	0	2 X	2 C	2 X	Checklist for sustainability; reference list; glossary
Bertrand & Solis "Evaluating HIV/AIDS Prevention Projects: A Manual for Nongovernmental Organizations". MEASURE. http://www.cpc.unc.edu/measure/publications/pdf/ms-04-10.pdf. Accessed April 6, 2005.	4 - overview pdf	NGOS working on HIV/AIDS programs	2	2	2	0	0	2 X	2	2 X	1	2	0	0	2 T X	2 T	2	0	2	0	0	List of indicators; appendix on sampling, overview of illustrative HIV/ AIDS programs w/objectives, references

Reference	Format	Audience																			Notes
(1999) "A Guide for First Nations on Evaluating Health Programs." Health Canada. http://www. hc-sc.gc.ca/fnihb-dgspni/fnihb/ bpm/hfa/transfer_publications/ evaluating_health_programs.pdf. Accessed April 21, 2005.	4 - overview pdf	First Nation communities	2	2	0	2 X	0	2	0	1	1	0	0	0	0	0	0	2	0	0	
"Community How to Guide on Evaluation." NHTSA. http:// www.nhtsa.dot.gov/people/injury/ alcohol/community%20guide…. Accessed March 28, 2005.	4 - overview pdf	Program managers in underage drinking prevention programs	1	2	2	0	1	2 C	0	0	0	1	0	1	1	1	1	1	1	0	List of sample survey and focus group questions for underage drinking programs
(2004) "Evaluation Guidebook for Small Agencies": Treasury Board of Canada Secretariat: http://www.tbs-sct.gc.ca/eval/dev/ sma-pet/guidelines/guidebook_ e.pdf. Accessed April 27, 2005.	4 - overview pdf	Small Canadian agencies required by treasury board to submit	2	2	2	2 L R X	1	2 C	2 L	0	2	0	0	2 R	1	1	2 C	1 C R	2 C	1	Appendix on questionnaire development, glossary
(March 2004) "Programme Manager's Planning Monitoring & Evaluation Toolkit." UNFPA. http://www.unfpa.org/monitoring/ toolkit.htm. Accessed April 26, 2005.	4 - overview pdf	Program managers in reproductive health	2	3 R	2 R	1	2 R T	3 R T	2 R	0	1	1	1	2	2	3 R	0	2 R	2 C T	2	Glossary, reference lists
(2003) "Project Evaluation toolkit." University of Tasmani. http://www.utas.edu.au/pet/pdf/ fullcontents/pdf. Accessed April 21, 2005.	4 - overview pdf	Program managers	2	2	0	2 L R W X	0	2 W	2 L R W X	0	0	1	2 W	1 L R	2 W	0	0	2 W	1	2	Overview of data storage considerations

Literature Review Matrix — Evaluation Handbooks

Code: 0=Not mentioned, 1=Mentioned, little detail, 2=Topic covered, 3=Extensive discussion of topic. L=Link to other source, C=Checklist, R=References, T=Table/chart/picture, W=Worksheet, X=Examples

Reference	Format/ design	Target population	Overview/description	Why, how, when & for	Types of eval.	Decision-making tree	Logic models	Objectives/indicators	Stakeholders	Data collection	Software for data	Eval questions	Ethical considerations	Budget/resources	Quantitative analysis	Qualitative analysis	Data quality/standards	Interpretation/action	Reporting results	Outside evaluators	Pitfalls/FAQs/barriers	Other
Baker, et al. (2000) "An Evaluation Framework for Community Health Programs." CDC & Center For the Advancement of Community Based Public Health. http://www.cdc.gov/eval/evalcbph.pdf. Accessed March 24, 2005.	4 - overview pdf	CBOs	3 R	2 T W X	2	1	2 W X	2 W X	3 T W X	1 W	0	0	0	1	1	1	1	2 W X	2 T W	0	0	Glossary;
Chinman, M, Imm, P & Wandersman, A (2004) "Getting to Outcomes 2004: Promoting Accountability Through Methods and Tools for Planning, Implementation, and Evaluation." Rand Health. http://www.rand.org/pubs/technical_reports/2004/RAND_TR101.pdf. Accessed April 11, 2005.	4 - overview pdf	Program managers with alcohol, tobacco & drug programs	2	2	2	0	2 X	2	0	2 L R T	0	2 T	2	0	1	1	0	2	0	0	0	Chapter on sustainability

Citation	Format	Audience	Ratings (left to right)	Notes
Farell, K, Kratzmann M, McWilliam, S, Robinson, N, Saunders, S, Ticknor, J & White, K (2002) "Evaluation made Very easy, Accessible and Logical (EVAL)." http://www.acewh.dal.ca/eng/reports/EVAL.pdf.	4 - overview pdf	Non-profits	1, 1, 2, 0, 2 L X, 1, 2, 2 L, 2 L, 1 L, 1 L, 1, 0, 1, 1, 0, 2, 0, 0, 0	Glossary; list of sample evaluations by project focus; links to other on-line resources
Mizell, L (2003) "Program Evaluation, A Primer, 2nd ed". Http://www.leemizell.com/freedocs/primer_free.pdf. Accessed March 28, 2005	4 - overview pdf	Program managers & staff who are new to evaluation	2, 2 L, 2, 1 T, 1, 2, 0, 0, 2, 0, 2, 0, 1, 0, 1, 0, 1, 2 L, 1	Glossary; list of references
Molund & Schill (2004) "Looking Back, Moving Forward. Sida Evaluation Manual". Sida. http://www.sida.se/content/1/c6/02/56/24/SIDA3753en_mini.pdf. Accessed April 4, 2005.	4 - overview pdf	Sida staff involved in development interventions	2, 2, 2, 0, 0, 2 C, 0, 2 C, 0, 2 C, 0, 0, 2 C, 0, 2 C, 2 C T, 2 C, 0	Glossary
Suvedi, M, Hainze, K & Ruonavaara, D (Dec 1999) "How to Conduct Evaluation of Extension Programs." ANRECS Center for Evaluative Studies, East Lansing. http://www.canr.msu.edu/evaluate/AllTextMaterial/evaluation%20-manual%202000.html. Accessed April 21, 2005.	4 - overview pdf	Extension program directors	1, 2, 1, 0, 1, 1, 2, 0, 0, 0, 0, 0, 0, 2 X, 1, 1, 2, 2, 0, 0	
Donnelly, et al. (eds.) (1997) "Who Are the Question-Makers? A Participatory Evaluation Handbook". Office of evaluation and strategic planning (OESP), United Nations Development Programme. New York. http://www.undp.org/eo/documents/who.htm. Accessed April 21, 2005.	5 - overview html	UNDP program managers		

Literature Review Matrix — Evaluation Handbooks

Code: 0=Not mentioned, 1=Mentioned, little detail, 2=Topic covered, 3=Extensive discussion of topic. L=Link to other source, C=Checklist, R=References, T=Table/chart/picture, W=Worksheet, X=Examples

Reference	Format/design	Target population	Overview/description	Why, how, when & for	Types of eval.	Decision-making tree	Logic models	Objectives/indicators	Stakeholders	Data collection	Software for data	Eval questions	Ethical considerations	Budget/resources	Quantitative analysis	Qualitative analysis	Data quality/standards	Interpretation/action	Reporting results	Outside evaluators	Pitfalls/FAQs/barriers	Other
Kantor & Kendall-Tackett (eds.) (Dec 2000) "A Guide to Family Intervention and Prevention Program Evaluation". US Air Force family advocacy program. http://www.fourh.umn.edu/ evaluation/family/default.html. Accessed April 6, 2005.	5 - overview html	Program managers in family advocacy projects	1	2	2 R	W	2 R T W X	1	2	2 R X	0	2	1	1	0	0	2	0	0	2	0	Cost analysis chapter
"Guide to Project Evaluation: A Participatory Approach". Public Health Agency of Canada. http://www.phac-aspc.gc.ca/ph-sp/phdd/resources/guide/index. htm#CONTENTS. Accessed April 11, 2005.	5 - overview html	Those working on participatory evaluations																				
AROW (Action & Research Open Web). "Program Evaluation." http://www2.fhs. usyd.edu.au/arow/o/m06/m06. htm. Accessed March 25, 2005.	5 - overview html	Beginners who want brief overview of evaluation	2	0	2	0	0	0	0	2 R W	0	2 R	2	2	1	0	2	0	2	0	0	

Reference	Format	Audience	Ratings (left → right)	Comments
BJA (bureau of justice assistance), Center for Program Evaluation. "Guide to Program Evaluation." http://www.ojp.usdoj.gov/BJA/evaluation/guide/index.htm. Accessed April 6, 2005.	5 - overview html	Managers of youth justice programs	1, L, L, T, L, 0, L, 0, L, L(X), L, 0, L, 0, 0, L, L, 0, 0, 0	
CSAP. "Building a Successful Prevention Program: Step 7, Evaluation Center for Substance Abuse Prevention" University of Nevada, Reno. http://casat.unr.edu/bestpractices/eval.htm. Accessed April 11, 2005.	5 - overview html	Managers of prevention programs	2, 2, 2(W), 2, 2, 2(X), 2(X), 0, 2(X), 0, 2, 2, 2, 0, 2, 2, 2, 2(C), 2, 0	Glossary
UNESCO. "Evaluation Manual." http://www.unesco.org/ios/eng/evaluation/tools/outil_e.htm. Accessed April 6, 2005.	5 - overview html	Those who just need brief outline of eval.	2, 1, 0, T, 1, 0, 2, 1(R,X), 0, 1, 1, 0, 0, 1, 0, 1, 0, 0	Excellent glossary with examples and characteristics; guide to questionnaire writing
University of Sydney, Australia, Action & Research Open Web. "Program Evaluation." http://ww2.fhs.usyd.edu.au/arow/o/m06/m06.htm. Accessed March 25, 2005.	5 - overview html	General public, students, etc.	1, 1, 2, 0, 1, 2, 2(R), 0, 1(R), 2, 1, 1, 1(R), 1, 1, 0, 0	
APDIME. "Toolkit, Version 2.0: Resources for HIV/AIDS Program Managers." http://www.synergyaids.com/apdime/mod_5_eval/eval_index.htm. Accessed March 30, 2005.	6 - overview in online interactive format	Beginners: program managers working on HIV/AIDS	1, 2, 1, 0, 2(L,T), 1, 2(L), 0, 0, 2, 2(L), 1(L), 2(L,T), 2, 1, 0	List of indicator resources (databases, etc); lots of links to other guides & resources

Literature Review Matrix — Evaluation Handbooks

Code: 0=Not mentioned, 1=Mentioned, little detail, 2=Topic covered, 3=Extensive discussion of topic. L=Link to other source, C=Checklist, R=References, T=Table/chart/picture, W=Worksheet, X=Examples

Reference	Format/design	Target population	Overview/description	Why, how, when & for	Types of eval.	Decision-making tree	Logic models	Objectives/Indicators	Stakeholders	Data collection	Software for data	Eval questions	Ethical considerations	Budget/resources	Quantitative analysis	Qualitative analysis	Data quality/standards	Interpretation/action	Reporting results	Outside evaluators	Pitfalls/FAQs/barriers	Other
CSN National Children's Center for Rural and Agricultural Health and Safety (1997) "Evaluation Guidebook for Community Youth Safety Programs, 2nd ed." CSN, HRSA. http://research.marshfieldclinic.org/children/Resources/evaluation_guidebook.pdf. Accessed April 26, 2005.	7 - segment - definition of eval. & 2 types	Those involved in community youth safety programs	2	2	2 T	0	0	1	0	0	0	0	0	0	0	0	0	0	0	0	0	
University of Wisconsin, Extension. "Enhancing Program Performance with Logic Models." http://www.uwex.edu/ces/lmcourse/#.	7 - segments in online interactive format	Program managers	1	2	1	0	3 C L R T W	2 W X	1	2 L	0	2	0	0	1	1	0	0	0	0	0	
							W															
Government of Canada, Human Resources Development. "Evaluation Tool kit Series." http://www11.hrdc-drhc.gc.ca/pls/edd/toolkit.list.	7 - segments in pdf series	Aboriginal Human Resource Development Agreement holders	3	2	2	0	0	2	0	1	0	2	0	0	2	0	2 R X	0	0	0	0	

Source	Format	Audience																				Notes
USAID Evaluation publications site. http://www.dec.org/usaid_eval/#toc.	7 - segments in pdf series	Project directors working for USAID	2 L R	2	1	0	0	2	0	1	1	1	0	1	1	2	2	1	1	0	0	Information split between several 'Tips' documents.
"Evaluation Tipsheets." PennState, College of Agricultural Sciences Cooperative Extension & Outreach. http://www.extension.psu.edu/evaluation/titles.html.	7 - series of tip sheets on evaluation	Anyone working on evaluation projects																				
CDC & University of Texas-Houston Health Science Center, School of Public Health & TX department of Health. "Practical Evaluation of Public Health Programs Workbook." http://www.cdc.gov/eval/workbook.pdf. Accessed March 24, 2005	7 - workbook in pdf	Workbook that went along with webcast from CDCat one point	1	2	0	0	1	1	1	1	1	0	0	1	0	1	1	1	0	1		Framework for program evaluation;
Tang, H (Dec 2004) "Local Program Evaluation Planning Guide." California Department of Health Services: Tobacco Control Section. http://www.dhs.ca.gov/tobacco/documents/EvalPlanningGuide2004.pdf. Accessed April 21, 2005.	7 - workbook in pdf	Those working on tobacco control programs	0	0	1	0	3 C X	1	2 X	0	0	0	0	0	0	2	0	2	0	2		Lots of case studies
Microsoft & Npower. "Npower Program Evaluation Toolkit." http://www.npower.org/tools/directory/eval/. Accessed March 23, 2005.	8 - intermediate level guides html	IT personnel	1 L R	0	0	1 X	1	0	2 L R	0	1 L R X	0	1 R	1 R	0	0	1 R	0	0	0		

Literature Review Matrix — Evaluation Handbooks

Code: 0=Not mentioned, 1=Mentioned, little detail, 2=Topic covered, 3=Extensive discussion of topic. L=Link to other source, C=Checklist, R=References, T=Table/chart/picture, W=Worksheet, X=Examples

Reference	Format/ design	Target population	Overview/ description	Why, how, when & for	Types of eval.	Decision-making tree	Logic models	Objectives/indicators	Stakeholders	Data collection	Software for data	Eval questions	Ethical considerations	Budget/resources	Quantitative analysis	Qualitative analysis	Data quality/standards	Interpretation/action	Reporting results	Outside evaluators	Pitfalls/FAQs/barriers	Other
Baker, JL (2000) "Evaluating the Impact of Development Projects on Poverty: A Handbook for Practitioners." World Bank. http://siteresources.worldbank.org/INTISPMA/Resources/Impact-Evaluation-Handbook-English-/impact1.pdf (also impact2-6.pdf). Accessed April 6, 2005.	8 - intermediate level guides in pdf series	Practitioners of impact evaluation in developing countries	2 R	2 T W	2	0	0	2	0	2 T	0	2	0	2 X	1	1	2	0	2	2	0	Lots of case studies; examples of other impact evaluations in developing countries
Burroughs, W. (2000) "Measuring the Difference: Guide to Planning and Evaluating Health Information Outreach." National Library of Medicine. http://nnlm.gov/evaluation/guide/. Accessed March 28, 2005.	8 - intermediate level guides pdf	Health information outreach project personnel	2 R	2 T W	2 R T	0	0	2 R W X	1	2 T W	1	1	0	1	2 X	2	2	2	2 R	0	0	Table of resources needed for eval. types; info. on t-tests, ANOVA, regression, etc.; appendices on objectives, planning, surveys,

Citation	Format	Audience																		Notes
LaFond & Brown (March 2003) "A Guide to Monitoring and Evaluation of Capacity-Building Interventions in the Health Sector in Developing Countries." MEASURE & USAID. MEASURE evaluation manual series, no. 7. http://www.cpc.unc.edu/measure/publications/pdf/ms-03-07.pdf. Accessed March 6, 2005.	8 - intermediate level guides pdf	Those involved in capacity-building interventions in developing countries	2	2	0	2 T X	0	2 X	1	2 L T	0	0	0	0	0	0	2	0	0	0	Summaries at end of each section; list of indicators; links to data measurement tools; overall checklist
Lana (1993) "Understanding Evaluation: The Way to Better Prevention Programs." Department of Education Muraskin. http://www.ed.gov/PDFDocs/handbook.pdf. Accessed March 25, 2005.	8 - intermediate level guides pdf	Those performing activities under drug-free schools act & required to do eval.	2	2	2	0	0	2	0	2 X	0	2 X	1	0	2	2 X	0	2	0	2	Fictitious case study used throughout guide as an example;
Rehle et al. "Evaluating Programs for HIV/AIDS Prevention and Care in Developing Countries: A Handbook for Program Managers and Decision makers." FHI. http://hivinsite.ucsf.edu/inSite?page=li-11-01#s2x. Accessed March 30, 2005.	8 - intermediate level guides pdf	Program managers working on HIV/AIDS projects	0	1	2 R T	1 T	2 R X	0	2 R T X	1	2 R	1	3	1	2	2	1	0	2	0	List of indicators; chapters on validity of self-reported data, sampling, impact & cost-effectiveness evals., AVERT model for impact
"Handbook on Monitoring and Evaluating for Results;" UNDP Evaluation office. http://stone.undp.org/undpweb/eo/evalnet/docstore3/yellowbook/documents/full_draft.pdf. Accessed April 11, 2005	8 - intermediate level guides pdf	General program managers	0	1	1	0	2 W	2	1	0	1	2	1	0	3	1	1	0	2	0	Sample surveys, other tools in appendices

Literature Review Matrix — Evaluation Handbooks

Code: 0=Not mentioned, 1=Mentioned, little detail, 2=Topic covered, 3=Extensive discussion of topic.   L=Link to other source, C=Checklist, R=References, T=Table/chart/picture, W=Worksheet, X=Examples

Reference	Format/design	Target population	Overview/description	Why, how, when & for	Types of eval.	Decision-making tree	Logic models	Objectives/indicators	Stakeholders	Data collection	Software for data	Eval questions	Ethical considerations	Budget/resources	Quantitative analysis	Qualitative analysis	Data quality/standards	Interpretation/action	Reporting results	Outside evaluators	Pitfalls/FAQs/barriers	Other
Callor et al. (2000) "Community-Based Project Evaluation Guide." University of Arizona. http://ag.arizona.edu/fcs/cyfernet/cyfar/stst_guide.pdf. Accessed April 6, 2005.	8 - intermediate level guides pdf	Those working on CFAR projects. Not for beginners to eval.	2 X	2	1	0	2 X	0	1	0	0	1	0	0	1	0	0	0	1	0	0	5-tiered approach, references
CDC (1999) "Framework for Program Evaluation in Public Health." MMWR, 48(RR-11). http://www.cdc.gov/eval/framework.htm. Accessed March 24, 2005.	8 - intermediate level guides pdf	Public Health professionals	1	2 T	0	0	2 X	2	2 T	1 T	0	0	0	1	1	1	2 T	1	2 C	1	1	Framework for program evaluation; continuing education activity; list of references
CDC, WHO, World Bank, Unicef, etc. (June 2004) "Monitoring & Evaluation Toolkit: HIV/AIDS, Tuberculosis and Malaria." http://www.who.int/hiv/pub/epidemiology/en/me_toolkit_en.pdf. Accessed April 4, 2005.	8 - intermediate level guides pdf	Those working at country level on M&E linked to HIV, TB or malaria programs	0	1	1	0	1 T	2 T X	0	0	0	1	0	0	1	1	1	0	1	0	2	References

Reference	Level / Format	Audience																	Notes
CDC. "Program Operations: Guidelines for STD Prevention. Program Evaluation." http://www.cdc.gov/std/program/progeval/TOC-Pgprogeval.htm. Accessed March 21, 2005.	8 - intermediate level guides pdf	Public Health personnel & program managers on STD programs	1	1	3 T	0	2 X	1	1	0	1	1	1	1	1	1	0	2	Glossary; reference List
Shared Intelligence (2002) "Evaluation in the National Council — ELWa: A Step-by Step Guide." ELWa (Education and learning Wales). http://www.elwa.org/uk/elwaweb/elwa.aspx?pageid=2065. Accessed April 21, 2005.	8 - intermediate level guides pdf	ELWa program managers	2	1	2	0	T	1	2	0	2	2 R	1	1 X	1	2	2	0	Case-study examples, glossary, appendices on other eval. paradigms and quantitative analysis (anova, chi2, t-test, etc.)
Canadian International Development Agency. "How to Perform Evaluations." http://www.acdi-cida.gc.ca/cida_ind.nsf/49d9f10330ed2bb4852567.... Accessed March 28, 2005.	8 - intermediate overview in pdf series	CIDA managers working on development projects	0	1	0	0	0	2 C	1	0	1 C X	1	0	2 C X	1	2 C	2 C	0	
City of Ottawa. "A Program Evaluation Toolkit." http://ottawa.ca/city_services/grants/toolkit/index_en.shtml. Accessed March 25, 2005.	9 - how-to guide for purchase ($40)	Managers and staff in CBOs who want to conduct in-house eval.																	
"Community Health Worker Evaluation Toolkit: Increasing the Quality and Quantity of Community Health Worker Program Evaluations." University of Arizona Rural Health Office and College of Public Health.	9 - how-to guide for purchase ($49)	Community health workers																	Tips for grant-writing, logic model development,

Literature Review Matrix — Evaluation Handbooks

Code: 0=Not mentioned, 1=Mentioned, little detail, 2=Topic covered, 3=Extensive discussion of topic. L=Link to other source, C=Checklist, R=References, T=Table/chart/picture, W=Worksheet, X=Examples

Reference	Format/design	Target population	Overview/description	Why, how, when & for	Types of eval.	Decision-making tree	Logic models	Objectives/Indicators	Stakeholders	Data collection	Software for data	Eval questions	Ethical considerations	Budget/resources	Quantitative analysis	Qualitative analysis	Data quality/standards	Interpretation/action	Reporting results	Outside evaluators	Pitfalls/FAQs/barriers	Other
United Way of America (1996) "Measuring Program Outcomes: A Practical Approach." http://national.unitedway.org/outcomes/resources/mpo/.	9 - how-to guide for purchase ($5)	Health, human service and youth and family-serving agencies																				
Innonet (innovation network online). http://www.innonet.org. Accessed April 6, 2005.	9 - how-to in online interactive format	Those needed to design evaluation			2		3 W	2		2												
LTDI (Learning Technology Dissemination Initiative). "Evaluation Cookbook." http://www.icbl.hw.ac.uk/ltdi/cookbook/contents.html. Accessed March 30, 2005.	9 - online guide for lecturers in evaluation	Educators	0	2	2	0	1	0	0	2 R	1	0	0	0	1	1 R	0	1	1	0	0	
CDC, Division of adolescent and school health. "Handbook for Evaluating HIV Education." http://www.cdc.gov/HealthyYouth/publications/hiv_handbook/download.htm. Accessed April 6, 2005.	9 - overview of HIV education programs, brief guide on eval.	Program managers of HIV/AIDS education	2	2	0	0	0	2	0	2 W	1	2	2	0	0	3 W	0	2	3 X	3 W X	0	List of software for qualitative data; full booklets on qualitative data and on reporting evaluation results

																References
National funding collaborative on violence (June 2001) "Principles for Evaluating Comprehensive Community Initiatives." http://www.capablecommunity.com/pubs/NFCVP062001.pdf. Accessed April 6, 2005.	9 - professional evaluators	Professional evaluators	0	0	0	0	3	0	0	0	0	0	0	0	3	0	
(1997) "Evaluating Comprehensive Community Change." Report of the Annie E. Casey Foundation's March 1997 Research and Evaluation Conference.	9 - report that followed con-ference		0	0	1	0	1	1	1	0	1	0	0	1	0	0	
Clark, M & Sartorius, R (2004) "Monitoring & Evaluation: Some Tools, Methods & Approaches." World Bank. http://lnweb18. worldbank.org/oed/oeddoclib. nsf/24cc3bb1f94ae.... Accessed April 21, 2005.	9 - review of a few tools for eval.	Those involved in evaluation	0	1	1	1	1	1	0	0	0	0	0	0	0	0	

Appendix 1
Data Collection Tools

Contents

In-depth Interviews

1. Clarify the purpose of the interview

Why are you doing an interview? What information do you hope to gain?

Program description:

_____

_____

_____

Purpose of evaluation:

_____

_____

_____

_____

Purpose of interviews:

_____

_____

_____

_____

_____

2. Determine staff responsibilities

- *Recruitment* – One person can generally handle calling and recruiting interviewees
- *Interviewers* – Usually one staff member can handle the interviews. If you intend to have more than three-four interviews, however, or if they will be scheduled close together, you may need to train more than one person to perform the interviews.
- *Transcriber* – Typing out a conversation that may have lasted 2 h can take over a full day. It is extremely important, however, that this be done, so make sure you have allotted time for someone on your staff to perform this job after each interview

Do not let more than a few days pass between the interview and the transcription — or the interviewer may forget details and not be able to help if there is a problem with the tape recording or something the transcriber doesn't understand.

3. *Select the respondents*

- Choose people who are opinion-leaders or who have valuable information or opinions that you wish to hear.
- There may be specific people you want to interview, such as local politicians, or there may just be a *type* of person you want to interview, such as physicians or people actively involved in community organizations.
- Ask potential respondents to participate well in advance of the interview
  - Whether you invite people by phone, by mail, or in person, give them a description of the program and the purpose of the interview
  - Explain what topics you will be asking about, and tell the person how long you expect the interview to last.
  - Mail a follow-up reminder a week or so before the interview, and include a list of questions or topics that will be discussed.
  - Call the person a day or two beforehand to remind them of the time and place.

	Interviewee Name & Title	Date/Time of interview	Interviewer name
	Phone/Address	Location of interview	Transcriber name
1			
2			
3			
4			
5			

4. Write the interviewer's guide

- Develop up to five or six *themes* and write several *potential* questions for each theme. The interviewer can then choose whichever question fits best with the flow of the conversation (or can make up new questions on the same theme)
- Use the 'funnel' effect, by starting with a very broad question and then progressively getting more specific. The broader questions help to build trust and to get the conversation going, so that you are more likely to get good answers for the sensitive or specific questions later on.

Southern Primary HealthCare Clinics Example	
Theme 1: Personal perspectives on cardiovascular disease and hypertension among clients	**Q1:** Do you think the problem of hypertension and CVD has increased or decreased over the past 5 years? **Q2:** Looking at statistics, it appears that not everyone in a community is at equal risk of hypertension. Would you say that is true? **Q3:** ...
Theme 2: Assessment of client knowledge	**Q1:** How would you describe the level of knowledge among your patients with regards to hypertension and cardiovascular disease? **Q2:** Would you say the level of knowledge among patients about hypertension and CVD is higher or lower than 5 years ago? **Q3:** ...
Theme 3: ...	**Q1:** ...

The interviewers must be fully informed of the purpose of the interview and what information is hoped to be obtained. Only then can he or she decide when to allow a conversation to 'drift' away from the set questions (because useful information is being discussed, even though it wasn't planned for), or when to cut off a stream of thought and return to the written themes. In all cases, the interviewer must allow sufficient time to hit all of the themes (though not necessarily all of the questions within each theme).

Facilitator's Guide — In-depth Interview

Project name: _____

Goal of the interview: _____

_____

Respondent's Name: _____

Interviewer's Name: _____

Date/Time of Interview: _____

Location of Interview: _____

Reminders for the facilitator:

The interview should flow as a casual conversation would

- Greet the person warmly. Make sure the respondent and yourself have something to drink and a snack.
- Confirm that the respondent is comfortable.
- Start off with a minute or two of 'small talk'—ask about the respondent's day, etc.

Explain purpose of interview

- Begin by reviewing the purpose of the interview
- Make sure the respondent knows that you are interested in their opinions on the subject, even if their comments do not directly answer one of your questions.

Maintain neutrality

- Be very careful not to allow your own opinions to show, or to encourage certain types of comments

Use active listening

- Make appropriate eye contact with respondent.
- Nod, and offer confirmatory remarks such as 'yes, that's interesting' to encourage conversation.
- You should not to any more than about 10% of the talking. Talk only as much as required to keep the conversation going and to keep the respondent comfortable.

Be the time keeper

- Pay attention to time and decide when you need to steer the conversation towards themes you haven't covered yet.
- Do *not* let the time run over what was promised at the beginning.

Take notes

- Make notes on a separate pad of paper. Along with comments said, include notes about the environment, any disturbances that may happen, the mood or expressions of the respondent, and other relevant information.
- Write down your general impressions from the interview at the end, after you have thanked the person and ended the interview.

Clock time for start of interview: _____

Interviewer—try to cover each theme listed. The questions by each theme are to serve as a guide. You may use them as you deem appropriate. You do not need to cover the themes in order. If other themes come up that you deem as relevant, feel free to explore them as long as you leave adequate time to cover the themes listed here.

Theme 1:	Q1:
	Q2:
	Q3:
Theme 2:	Q1:
	Q2:
	Q3:
Theme 3:	Q1:
	Q2:
	Q3:
Theme 4:	Q1:
	Q2:
	Q3:
Theme 5:	Q1:
	Q2:
	Q3:

Clock time for end of interview: _____

Include Interviewer comments in notes from interview (*general feelings about interview, any disturbances or circumstances that may have affected the interview, or other information relevant to interpreting the answers given*).

5. Ethics and confidentiality

- Informed consent
  - See Chapter 3 for information on informed consent, and Worksheet #4 for a sample consent form.
  - Have two copies of the informed consent available, so you can keep one and give the respondent a copy.
- Confidentiality
  - If the session will be tape recorded, where will the tape be stored? Will the respondent's name be kept in a record somewhere, and if so—who will have access to that record?
  - Plan for the long term. Remember that staff may quit or leave your project and others may join, so have a system in mind for which staff member will have access to any records with participants' names or personal information.

6. Prepare for the interview

- Ensure that you have a private, comfortable location for the interview. It should be an area that no other people will enter into during the interview, both to prevent interruptions and to protect the respondent's privacy.
- If the interview will be over lunch, you should provide lunch for the respondent. Otherwise, have a snack and something to drink on hand.
- If you decide to tape record the session, test the recorder to make sure it works beforehand and ensure that you have enough memory or blank tapes and enough battery power for the entire session.

7. Conduct the interview

- Introductions
  - Begin the interview as you would a conversation with someone you just met. Introduce yourselves, and chat a minute or two about backgrounds, the weather, the traffic, or whatever.
  - Make sure the respondent has something to drink.
  - Review again the purpose of the interview and the topics that will be discussed.
  - If you have decided to tape record, ask for permission to turn the tape on. Review issues of privacy and confidentiality, and tell the respondent how the information will be used and how the notes and/or tape from the session will be stored.
- Obtain informed consent
  - Read or have the respondent read the informed consent form.
  - Answer any questions, keep the signed copy and give the respondent his or her own copy.

- Interviewing
  - Start with some of the broad questions from theme 1 on the interviewer's guide. By the time you move on to theme 2, the respondent should already be doing 90% of the talking.
  - Conduct the interview as if it were a casual conversation.
  - Lead the respondent back if the conversation strays too far, but try to avoid interrupting or disrupting the flow of the conversation.
  - Use note-taking as a tool to introduce pauses or short silences into the conversation. These can help the respondent think through an answer or hit upon something else he or she wanted to say.
- Concluding
  - Thank the respondent warmly, and explain again how the information will be used to improve services.
- Wrapping up
  - Review your notes and tape and write up a summary of the session immediately afterwards. Write down you feelings about the interview and the information obtained. It is important to do this while your memory is still fresh, so that gaps in the notes or tape can be filled in immediately.
  - A transcript of the session or copy of the summary should be sent to the respondent to verify the accuracy of the information and to show that the results will be used. It is perfectly acceptable to highlight areas where more information would have been more useful or to include an additional question or two. After having more time to think, the respondent may have more information to give.

8. Tips for overcoming roadblocks

Difficulties in scheduling or getting people to agree to be interviewed.

- Plan in advance. Give the person several weeks notice to make sure you get on his or her calendar early.
- Be flexible. Be ready to schedule evening or weekend times if they work out better for the person. Also be willing to travel to a convenient in-between location (it's not wise to meet in the person's own office, however, as the likelihood of getting interrupted by phone calls or other distractions is high!)
- Be open and sincere. Emphasize the public health nature of your project, and how the interview will ultimately help you improve programs that will benefit the community. Be open about what the interview is about, and why you are doing it. The more you can interest the person in the program or topic, the more likely he or she will be to agree to be interviewed.

- Go in person. It's a lot easier to refuse an invitation that is sent over email or regular mail than it is over the phone or in person. For very busy people, contact their secretaries and put yourself on their calendar. Send the email or postal mail invitation (personalized, and with an explanation of the program) just ahead of the date of your meeting so they have an idea of what you're talking about when you show up to ask them in person.

Dealing with difficult interviews

Respondent is reluctant to answer questions, or gives only short answers

- Return to a broad, easy question. An example might be, 'Some of our clients seem to think (X). Would you agree with that?'
- Ask the respondent about what they have seen or observed in relation to the topic you are discussing.
- Encourage answers through 'active listening'—nod, be enthusiastic and interested in the answers, and rephrase statements to ensure clarity and show that you are paying attention.

Respondent is suspicious of questions, or refuses to answer many questions

- Stay with non-sensitive, easy questions until the respondent starts opening up and offering more detailed information on his or her own.
- If the interview is being taped, offer to shut off the tape.
- Repeat the fact that confidentiality will be taken seriously, and inform the respondent that you can send a transcript of all notes for his or her approval before they are used in any report.
- As a last resort, you can keep the interview to only broad questions and ask the respondent if he or she would return for a follow-up interview. Before the second interview, send the respondent the summary from the first interview and ask for comments to show that you are taking the process seriously.

Respondent frequently strays from the topic

- Quite often this is a good thing and is exactly what you want to have happen. Sometimes, however, a person may stray too far too frequently.
- Try seizing on some small detail of what they are saying and relate it back to one of your questions or a previous comment of theirs that *was* on target.
- Take a moment to review the themes that you have already covered before asking the next question. That may help to realign the respondent with the desired flow of the conversation and help to keep things roughly on track.

Group Interviews

1. Clarify the purpose of the group interview

Why are you doing a group interview? What information do you hope to gain? Keep this purpose close at hand as you prepare for and carry out the group interview.

Program description:

_____

_____

_____

Purpose of evaluation:

_____

_____

_____

Purpose of group interviews:

_____

_____

_____

_____

2. Determine staff responsibilities

- *Overall coordinator*—schedules meeting with the rest of the staff working on the group interview and ensures that deadlines are met; trains facilitators and note-takers; completes work plan; prepares facilitator guide
- *Logistics*—Secures a room for the interviews; orders food or buys snacks and drinks; ensures there are adequate name tags, blank envelopes and pens for participants; tests tape recorder and ensures there is enough memory or blank tape and battery power for duration of group interviews; sends a letter and/or calls participants to remind them of the date, time & location; copies final summary and mails a copy to each participant.
- *Recruitment*—coordinates recruitment of participants; screens participants and explains purpose of group interview; acquires contact information for those who agree to participate; reports on progress of recruitment to coordinator on deadlines set by coordinator.
- *Facilitator*—conducts group interviews; reviews results and helps to write summary of group discussion after each group interview
- *Note-taker*—takes notes during group interview; assists facilitator as needed; reviews notes and helps to write summary of group discussion immediately after each group interview
- *Transcriber*—types out full transcript of the group interview discussion from audio tapes or notes.

3. Select participants

- A group interview should involve people who are similar to each other. You will likely have to hold several group interviews to hear from all the different groups you want to be represented.
- Make sure to separate groups of people who may act more dominant than others, or if the experiences of each are too different.

Group Interview Composition Tips:

Keep groups that are likely to be perceived as dominant over other groups separate. For example, you may want to have different groups for:

- Men and women
- People of different ages
- Doctors and nurses
- General workers and administrators

Depending on the type of questions you are asking, some groups may not feel comfortable answering around groups that may hold different opinions. For example, you may need to separate:

- City dwellers from rural dwellers
- People of different racial or ethnic backgrounds
- Parents from non-parents
- Retired persons from working adults
- People with different educational levels
- People from different social classes

- Participants should be sent a written invitation, with the purpose of the group interview and a list of discussion questions to be asked, at least a week or two in advance
- Send a reminder note or telephone call a day or so before. Be sure to emphasize the public health aspect of your program, and how the group interview will ultimately improve the program and contribute to the community
- As recruitment can be a difficult and lengthy process, you should also decide how long you want to try to recruit people. If you are attempting to recruit a group of people who are typically very busy and perhaps unlikely to jump at the chance of joining a group interview (such as physicians or lawmakers), you may want to schedule an extra few weeks to make sure you get the number you want.
- Select days of the week and times for the group interviews when most people that you would ideally want to come would be able to make it. For example, if most people in your population are working adults, Monday morning would not be a very good time for a group interview.
- If you will be using the same facilitator or note taker for all group interviews, you should leave enough time between each group for a full summary to be

written up. It is **not** a good idea to finish all the groups before writing up summaries. The facilitator and note taker will likely have a hard time remembering one group from another by then. Summaries should be written, and the tapes transcribed, right after each group and before that facilitator and note-taker conduct another group.

Focus Group Planner

Group composition*	Date/Time	Facilitator
Staff in charge of recruiting	Location of group interview	Note-taker
1		
2		
3		
4		
5		
6		
7		
8		

Make sure to include the total number of people you would like to have in the group.

Southern Primary HealthCare Clinics Example		
Group composition	Date/Time	Facilitator
Staff in charge of recruiting	Location	Note-taker
1	12 Women from clinics 1, 2 & 3	Sat, May 28th / 3pm	Marsha
	Marsha	Clinic 1 conference room	Karen

Try to have female facilitators for groups with women, and males for groups with men, whenever possible.

4. Write the facilitators guide and train the facilitator to use it

- You should plan for no more than 1.5–2 h for the group interview. Some of that time will be spent on introductions and wrap-up, so make sure to take that into consideration when writing the questions to be asked. You want to leave time for the group to discuss topics that come up that are important but that you may not have thought of or wrote questions about.
- Write four-five main discussion questions that start very broad and easy and then get more specific. This will make it easier for people to get engaged, and mimics the natural flow of normal conversation. Group participants should do 90% of the talking.
- 'Prompt questions' can be written as a tool for the facilitator to help people understand the main question and get involved in answering it. The facilitator may or may not use the prompt questions, so make sure that any question you think **must** be covered is written as a main discussion question.
- Be careful that you do not **lead** the participants into giving a certain type of answer. Consider the following two discussion questions:

'How important do you think after-school programs are to solving the problem of kids not getting enough exercise?'	'Some people think offering after-school programs for kids may help them get enough exercise. What are your thoughts on that?'

- The first question could be considered 'leading'. It **assumes** that the participants think after-school programs are important ('How important do you think...'). It also assumes that people think there really is a problem with kids not getting enough exercise. Participants may not feel that way at all, but may be lead into saying they are by the phrasing of the question. The second question may allow people to really think through their answers, and give their true opinions.
- Make sure to write any special instructions to the facilitator for each question. If you want to make sure a question is asked a certain way, or tell the facilitator about examples he or she can use if people are confused, put this information in the guide.

Facilitator's Guide—Group Interview

Project name: _____

Goal of the group interview: _____

_____

Interviewer's Name: _____

Date/Time: _____

Location of group Interview: _____

Reminders for the facilitator:

Create a relaxed, friendly environment

- Greet people warmly. Talk about everyday topics while they are getting refreshments.
- Check in with people to make sure they are comfortable.

Ask follow-up questions

- Encourage discussion by asking spontaneous follow-up questions.
- Ask for clarity about any comment you are unsure about (or want more information about)
- Ask for examples or descriptions
- Avoid asking *why* after a comment, as it can put people on the defensive

Maintain neutrality

- Do not make comments that suggest you thought an answer was good or correct (do *not* make comments such as 'good answer', or 'good idea')
- Keep comments neutral, such as 'that's interesting', 'uh-huh' or 'OK, thanks for that comment'
- Be very careful not to allow your own opinions to show, or to encourage certain types of comments
- Ask if others in the group have a different point of view

Ensure balance in participation

- Sit next to dominant talkers, and across from shy people.
- Break eye contact with someone talking too much, or avoid eye contact with someone who has commented too frequently
- Make eye contact with shy people.
- Interrupt only rarely

Use active listening

- Look at people who are talking. Break eye contact only to write notes or to encourage someone who is rambling to end their comment.
- Nod to show you are understanding the comment
- Repeat statements occasionally to ensure you got it correct

Be the time keeper

- Do not expect the group to pay attention to time—they expect you to handle that job
- Be purposeful about telling the group you need to move on to the next topic. Offer that there may be time at the end for additional comments if people do not seem ready to move on.
- Do *not* let the time run over what was promised at the beginning.

Clock time for start of session: _____

*Add clock time from above to time in parenthesis for each section. Write down answer on each line. Do this **before** starting the group. Make sure to start each section by the time you wrote on the line.*

TIME	QUESTIONS	INSTRUCTIONS
(:05) _____	*Welcome*—thank people for coming. Offer that they help themselves to snacks & drinks, but that they *not be seated yet*. Pass around name tags & marker and ask for people to write first names only. Hand out blank envelopes and ask people to address one to themselves.	• May want to have few extra chairs near snack table for people to sit temporarily, until you are ready to seat them in circle.
	Seating—Help people get seated. **The facilitator should sit next to more talkative, dominant persons, and across from more shy persons**	
	Introduction—Introduce yourself & note-taker. Explain role of note-taker and purpose of focus group. Main point—what you hope to gain from focus group, how it will be used. Inform people of what time focus group will end.	
	Begin recording—tell people you will turn on the recorder.	• Leave tape recorder in clearly visible location for duration of talk
	Privacy—explain that real names will not be used in connection with the session or comments made. Explain how tapes & notes will be handled and stored to protect confidentiality.	
	Group introduction—Ask each person to introduce themselves using first name only.	
	Ground rules—	
	1) all answers are right answers, none are better or worse than any others.	
	2) the purpose is not to convince anyone else or argue. You want to get all opinions, and the group was picked so that people would have different thoughts & opinions from each other	
	3) very important that people state their *own* opinions. Do not answer based on what an 'average person' or 'someone in the community' might think, but what *they* themselves think	

4) all people in the group should be respectful of the time, and allow everyone to contribute equally. Ask that people help you ensure that everyone gets to talk.

5) Ask permission to interrupt if time is running short or if it important that you move on to another topic. Explain that you have certain topics you need to make sure are discussed.

6) Ask for agreement about the ground rules, and if there are questions.

Suggested follow-up questions: (:___)	**Question 1**	• Read bold question exactly. • Use follow-up questions if necessary, but keep to minimum. • Repeat any question as necessary
	_____	
Tell me more about that....	Possible follow-up or probing questions • •	
Can you describe...	•	
(:___)	**Question 2**	
What was it about....	_____	
If you could decide...	Possible follow-up or probing questions •	
Does anyone else...	•	
Imagine for a moment that... (:___)	**Question 3**	
	_____	
What are some ways that...	Possible follow-up or probing questions • •	

Can you give me an example of…	(:___)	***Question 4***
	___	
Would you agree or disagree that…		Possible follow-up or probing questions • •
Could you tell me of a situation where the opposite would be true…	(:___) ———	***Question 5***
		Possible follow-up or probing questions • •
	(:___) ___	Wrap-up **Is there anything else you would like to add?** What else would you like to say that you didn't get a chance to say during the talk? Any further comments?	• If time allows, revisit topics that were cut short • If time allows, can explain that they can mention topics that were not discussed that they wanted to bring up.
	(:___)	Thank participants for coming. Hand out thankyou gifts. Explain that a brief summary of the findings will be sent to them using the envelope they filled out.	

Southern Primary HealthCare Example		
Clock time at start of session: <u>5:30pm</u>		
Suggested follow-up questions: Tell me more about that…. Can you describe… What was it about….	(:10) <u>5:40pm</u> (:25) <u>5:55pm</u>	***Question 1*** I'd like you all to think about some commercials for food you've seen lately. What are some food ads you saw on TV, in a magazine, or somewhere else that you remember? Possible follow-up or probing questions • Do you remember the last time you saw an advertisement for snack food? What was the ad for? • Can anyone remember an ad they saw recently for healthy food? ***Question 2*** Possible follow-up or probing questions •	• Read bold question exactly. • Use follow-up questions if necessary, but keep to minimum. • Repeat any question as necessary

- The times in parenthesis to the left of the questions show the maximum amount of time that should have passed when the facilitator moves onto that question. The facilitator should add that number to the clock time at the beginning of the session, so that the clock time for when the next question *must* be started is beside each question. In the example above, it was decided that only 10 min should be spent on introductions, and an additional 15 min or less spent on question #1. The facilitator fills in the clock time when he or she starts (5:30pm in this case), then adds the numbers in parenthesis to get the clock time to start each question (Question 1 must start at 5:40pm, question 2 by 5:55pm, etc).
- The facilitator should allow the conversation to drift to important topics that were not planned for, but that are useful to the goals of the group discussion. However, the facilitator must still be mindful of the time so that all questions can be addressed.
- The note-taker should be able to serve as a 'backup' facilitator. This person should write down the names of all participants, as well as a 'map' of where they are seated (so they can refer to their map to remember people's names as the discussion progresses). During the conversation, the note-taker should make notes not only about what is said, but also the mood, tone, and expressions of the person making comments.

Characteristics of a good facilitator:
- ❑ **Engaging** — able to keep lively group atmosphere going
- ❑ **Active listener** — encourages open discussion, rephrases comments for clarity
- ❑ **Dynamic** — able to respond to different group personalities and situations
- ❑ **Flexible** — can decide when to allow the conversation to stray to a different topic
- ❑ **Patient** — allows time for people to think through their answers

5. Ethics and confidentiality

- Have all participants sign an informed consent before beginning the group interview.
- Include information about the session being tape recorded, and what will happen with the tape after the discussion.
- Mention that your project will keep all names and personal information private, but be sure to also state that you cannot guarantee that other participants will not talk about what they hear at the discussion once it is over (although you should strongly urge all participants to keep everything they hear private).

6. Prepare for the group interview

Checklist for preparations:

- ❑ Facilitator selected and trained
- ❑ Note-taker selected and trained
- ❑ Staff member prepared to transcribe notes/tape
- ❑ Copies of informed consent on hand
- ❑ Tape recorder tested and ready
- ❑ Several extra pens (for participants to fill out envelope & sign informed consent)
- ❑ Blank envelope ready for each participant to self-address (to be sent summary of results later)
- ❑ Quiet, well-lit, temperature controlled room selected with enough space to comfortably fit all people
- ❑ Sufficient blank tapes or memory ready in room for recording entire focus group
- ❑ Table for food and sufficient plates, cups, napkins, etc. ready in room (if applicable)
- ❑ Small tokens of appreciation ready (such as gift certificates, lunch voucher, etc)
- ❑ Name tags ready for all participants, facilitator & note taker (with marker for writing names)

For participants who are traveling in for the group interview

- ❑ Written reminder sent several days in advance, with date/time, purpose of activity & list of questions
- ❑ Telephone reminder 1–2 days in advance
- ❑ Bus tokens, reimbursements for taxi, parking vouchers, or other travel arrangements prepared (if applicable)

7. Conduct the group interview

- Do not seat everyone as they walk in, instead allow them to stand and chat around the drinks table. The note-taker should already be making observations at this point.
- The facilitator and note-taker together should pay attention to which people seem very loud or very talkative before the group even gets started. When people are seated, the facilitator and note-taker should seat themselves next to those talkative people.
- Start off with a warm welcome, and thank everyone for participating. Do brief introductions, and review the purpose of the group interview and what the information will be used for.
- Lay down the ground rules. These will be things like comments must be kept fairly short and to the point, that everyone must be allowed to voice his or her opinion, and that the facilitator may interrupt if is felt that the conversation is getting off track.
- Inform people that the tape recorder will be turned on. Leave the tape recorder in full view at all times. If the topic is sensitive, you may want to give participants the option of asking for the recorder to be turned off for certain comments. Review issues of privacy and confidentiality, explaining how the notes and/or tape will be stored after session and the fact that names will not be used in any reports or communication.
- Ask an easy and broad question at the beginning can help to start generating discussion. Group conversation will tend to be dominated by a few very vocal people, so once the conversation gets under way the facilitator should make sure everyone in the room has a chance to speak (tips about how to deal with overly talkative people are at the end of this section).

> It is important that the facilitator make it known from the beginning that there are no right or wrong answers to any questions, and that the program is not looking for people to answer in a particular way. The facilitator should tell the group that their opinions are what matter, so that they should feel free to express their views at all times.

- The note-taker in the room should make notes of the general demeanor of the people in the group, and should record who makes each comment.
- The facilitator should keep the group on target, but should also allow the conversation to go off on topics that were not planned but that may be helpful. If the group had started discussing a very interesting aspect of the topic, at the next lull in the conversation the facilitator may choose to hold off on asking the next pre-planned question and instead ask a question that would help the group probe the unexpected aspect more.
- At the end, the facilitator should ask for any additional comments, and then again thank the participants for their feedback.

- Checklist for *after* the interview:

  ❑ Facilitator & note-taker reviewed notes, wrote comments immediately following group interview
  ❑ Tapes were checked immediately after to ensure full discussion was recorded clearly
  ❑ Tapes and notes transcribed within 2 days of focus group
  ❑ Brief summary of results drafted & mailed to all participants with follow-up thank you letter

8. Tips for overcoming roadblocks

Difficulties in scheduling or getting people to participate.

- Select a time and location for the group interview that is easy and convenient for the members. Lunchtime often works well if the group interview will not run over an hour or so;
- If participants have to travel for the group interview, offer to give participants bus tokens, or reimbursement for their travel expenses;
- Offer drinks and snacks at the beginning of the group, or provide lunch if the group will be held at lunchtime;
- Make sure to explain why the group interview is being conducted, and how the information collected could have a positive impact on the program and the community;
- Offer small incentives for participation, such as a certificate for a free music CD or a $5 gift certificate from a local store;
- Offer to send participants with a brief summary of the findings, so they can see that the information was used;
- If you enlist participants ahead of time, send them each a card in the mail that has the address, time, date and purpose of the group interview. It is often helpful to include a list of the questions that will be discussed as well. Follow-up with a reminder phone call a day or two before.

Handling a difficult group.

- Person gives lengthy or irrelevant answers, and gets upset when the facilitator interrupts.
  - Enlist the group's help at the very beginning of any group interview by asking their permission to cut them off if necessary. Explain how important it is that you get through all the material, and how you want to make sure everyone can leave on time. Ask if they agree that the facilitator can interrupt comments that are too long or whenever time is running short and the group needs to go on to the next question. After giving permission, people will tend to be less aggressive when the facilitator does indeed cut them off.

- A few people are dominating the discussion
    - First try unspoken conversation tactics. Break eye contact with someone speaking too long, and avoid eye contact with people who have been dominating the conversation. If the facilitator and note-taker are seated beside the more dominant, talkative people (and therefore across from the less talkative ones), this is easier to do consistently. Use any small gap in the conversation (a person breaks to take a breath), to jump in with a 'well, that's interesting, let's hear what someone else has to say about that', or a similar comment. If the problem persists, tell the group that you feel that you are not hearing the opinions from everyone. Ask them for suggestions on how to ensure that everyone gets a chance to talk.
- People in the group appear bored or reluctant to answer, or are giving answers that don't follow the questions
    - The group may not understand the questions fully. Try rephrasing the question in a different way. It may also help to take a brief moment to review again the purpose of the group interview, and ask participants to give you examples of questions *they* think you should ask about the problem—you may find that they are the same or similar to what you have (just phrased differently). If the conversation is simply lagging or the group is not being very response, try to go back and ask a very broad, easy-to-answer question that people are likely to respond to. For example, 'If you could change one thing about (X), what would it be?" is a question that is easy and that everyone should be able to answer. Once the conversation picks up a bit, move back to the main questions.

Case Studies

1. Clarify the purpose of the case study

Case studies can have various purposes, including:

- Description. Case studies can be used to describe a typical or atypical experience, perspective, or activity. Can improve the understanding of a situation by adding details or can be used to illustrate extreme examples.
- Explanation. Case studies can also be used to explain how or why a program is working (or not working). They can test assumptions about the program activities, and in some cases can be used to build a case towards showing the program worked.

Program description:

_____

_____

_____

Purpose of evaluation:

_____

_____

_____

_____

Purpose of case studies:

_____

_____

_____

_____

_____

2. Determine staff responsibilities

- It is usually preferable to have just one person conduct a single case study. Each case study will likely include interviews, and may include direct observations and reviews of documents. The staff member responsible for putting together the case study must be competent at these activities (see the sections on interviews and observations for more information), and must have sufficient flexibility in their work schedules to allow them to follow up on information as needed.

3. Select the focus of the case studies

- Case studies can be done on individuals, businesses, situations, or any number of foci
- Most case study subjects are done through *purposive sampling*—which simply means the subject is selected on purpose for some reason. An example would be to select clients who reported having negative experiences with the project, to 'tell the story' of what happened and show how improvements can be made.

4. Prepare an Outline

- Draft a rough outline of what information you want in the case study. This will follow closely from the goals of conducting the case study.
- Write down a few ideas for where to start gathering information. Include names of people to interview, documents to search, online resources, and others.
- Information that you gain from the interviews, observations or documents may lead you new sources of information that you hadn't originally anticipated. It is important to continue to follow through with new sources and leads until you are satisfied that you have the complete story.

5. Ethics and Confidentiality

- Privacy and confidentiality can be particularly tricky with case studies, as the purpose of the activity is to gather information from many different sources about a single person, group, organization, or occurrence. When collecting information from individuals, informed consent should always be obtained and the purpose and scope of the case study explained
- All information collected should be kept in a secure location that is not accessible to those outside of the evaluation team. When reporting the case study, real names and personal identifiers (such as specific addresses, exact age, or other characteristics detailed enough to identify a person) should not be used unless the individual has given *explicit* (written) permission to be identified.

6. Gather information

- Writing a case study really is like doing detective work—you need to follow the clues as you find them. The three components mainly used in case studies are in-depth or group interviews, review of existing documents, and direct observations.

- The point of a case study is to tell a story from start to finish, with *many different perspectives*. You want the *full* story of what happened. While you will probably start by interviewing the person or group who are most central to the case study, you will also want to ask questions of others who were involved to fill out the story.

7. *Sort information & write case study*

- Information gained from case study data collection should be sorted and written up immediately, even as the case study progresses. After an initial interview, for example, the interview should be transcribed and 'themes' from the discussion noted. Subsequent interviews should then touch on those themes to try to discover patterns. Similar for observations and document reviews, key points, new perspectives, or surprising details should be noted immediately and then watched for during subsequent data collection. Some of these themes and notes may turn out to be insignificant, but others may clue you in to common patterns that will help you create the final story.
- The final case study should be written up so that it tells the story from beginning to end. Different perspectives should be included, as well as different possibilities for why something happened.

8. *Tips for Overcoming Roadblocks*

Evaluator bias.

- Before you even begin a case study, your evaluation team probably has some idea of how or why things happen in your program. It can be very difficult to overcome these preconceived notions when gathering information. Some tips that might help to remember:
  - Seek information from a variety of sources about each case study. Make sure to include people or sources who often disagree with your point of view or who are critical of the program. These sources are more difficult to reach (they are less likely to want to talk to you), but are an invaluable way to challenge your assumptions.
  - Write out beforehand what your best guess is for how or why whatever your case study is about happens. Then set out to *disprove* that guess. Ask questions and seek information that will show that you are wrong. If your assumptions were right, you won't be able to disprove them. If they were wrong, you will be sure to get the information to show that.

Surveys

1. Clarify the purpose of the survey

Why are you doing a survey? What information do you hope to gain?

Program description:

_____

_____

_____

Purpose of evaluation:

_____

_____

_____

_____

Purpose of survey:

_____

_____

_____

_____

_____

2. Determine staff responsibilities

- Conducting a survey requires a good bit of staff time and effort. Develop a plan of tasks, deadlines, and staff responsibilities with your evaluation team. The following tasks are usually involved in conducting a survey, and will need to be delegated to members of your evaluation team.

  - Selection & recruitment of respondents
  - Development of questionnaire
  - Ethics & confidentiality
  - Pilot testing & revision of questionnaire
  - Administering questionnaire
  - Coding & entering data

Task	Date Due	Person(s) Responsible	Notes

Southern Primary HealthCare Example			
Task	Date due	Person(s) responsible	Notes
Convene meeting with stakeholders	No later than May 10th	Marsha	
Eval team meeting to prioritize items for survey	May 11th	Marsha, Paul, Karen, Sam	Conference room
Meeting t decide on respondents, format, confidentiality	May 13th	Marsha, Paul	
Write questionnaire & cover sheet	May 18-25th	Marsha, Karen	
Pilot test & revise questionnaire	May 30-June 3rd	Clinic staff / Marsha, Sam	
Administer questionnaire	June 13th-August 5th	Clinic staff	Marsha will oversee
Code & enter data	August 8-19th	Sam	
Analyze data	August 17-31st	Paul	With assistance from state univ. student

3. Select & recruit participants

- Determine who your target population is for your survey. This is generally a population such as your program clients, patients at a clinic, students at a school, members of a particular community, or so on.

    - Quite often, your target population will be too large to survey all of the people in the population. If you cannot survey everyone, the best way to select who to survey is through a simple random sample.
    - Have your evaluation team review Chapter 3—sampling techniques—and decide on the best way to select a good sample of people for your survey.

- Determine the timing of your survey, and whether the same people will be surveyed more than once (as that could influence how much contact information you need from each respondent).

    - If the purpose is to collect information for an outcome evaluation, you will likely want to administer the survey at baseline and at least once again further into the program. If the purpose is to assess how respondents felt about some contact with your program (clinic visit, educational session, etc), you may want to administer the survey only once after they have completed the contact, or once before and once after the contact to compare results.
    - Decide whether the survey will be repeated in the future, and at what intervals. This may change later on, but having an idea up front can help write more appropriate questions.

4. Develop questionnaire

- Determine the format of the survey. There are several formats that your survey could be in—including interviewer-administered (asking questions face-to-face), telephone (asking questions over telephone), self-administered (handing participants paper questionnaire to fill out), mail (sending participants paper questionnaire to fill out), and internet-based (participants log onto website either from their own location or at a location you set up).

Survey formats			
Format	Advantages	Disadvantages	Best when:
Interviewer administered	• Can explain questions, ensure that they are filled out in order • If good rapport is built, can get more honest answers • More personal, often taken more seriously	• Need to have enough staff to conduct interviews • Depending on the questions, some people may be reluctant to answer in person • Fairly expensive—requires the most resources	• Questions are complex or there are many skip patterns (how a person answers one question affects which other questions are then asked)
Telephone survey	• Respondents don't need to be able to read or write to participate • Can reach remote people easily • Quick and inexpensive way of getting feedback	• Those without telephones are excluded (usually young people and those with low income) • Can be difficult to get good response rate • Becoming more difficult as people switch to cell phones (cannot get list of numbers)	• Questionnaire is short and simple • Can reach most target population by phone • Participants likely somewhat interested in survey topic
Mail survey	• Respondents can fill out questions in private • Gives time for people to think about their answers • Relatively easy & inexpensive	• Need address list for respondents • Hard to ensure response rate • Cannot control who completes questions or how they do it	• Questions are simple and easy to follow • Respondents have some interest in topic—likely to respond
Self-administered handout	• Typically high response rate • Quick and fairly easy • Inexpensive	• Respondents must be able to read & understand questions	• Respondents are readily available (finishing a program activity, visiting the clinic, etc)
Internet based	• Respondents can answer in privacy • Eliminates need for data-entry (answers can be automatically entered in database) • Quick and inexpensive way of getting feedback	• Respondents without access to internet are excluded (mostly older and low income) • Cannot control who completes questions • Requires someone capable of designing the survey on the web	• Questions are fairly complex or are very personal • Target population likely to have access to internet

- Write the questions. This is often more difficult than it would seem. Consider the following as you write your questions:
  - Wording. As with all data collection questions, be very careful the questions are not *leading*. The wording is very important to getting good information. Consider some of the following good and not-so-good examples of questions:

Leading question		Better question
'Research has shown that breastfeeding newborns for at least 3 months can improve their health in various ways. How long did you breastfeed your last child?'	→	'Did you breastfeed your last child?' (Followed by, 'How long did you breastfeed for?' if the answer is yes)
'How many times a day do you usually eat snack foods that are bad for your health?'	→	'How many times in an average day do you eat salty or sugary snack foods?'
'Do you think there is a need for after-school exercise programs that could decrease the rates of obesity, heart disease, and diabetes among the children?'	→	'Do you think there is a need for after-school exercise programs for children?'

- Skip patterns. A skip pattern is when you skip over certain questions based on the answer to previous questions. For example, if a respondent answered that they did not have any children, you would want to *skip* over any subsequent questions that asked for details about children. Self-administered questionnaires (mailed or in person) shouldn't have many skip patterns, and any that are there should be clearly labeled. Consider the following example:

4. Do you currently have any type of health insurance?

☐ Yes
☐ No (*Skip to Question #6*)

5. Check all of the following types of insurance that you currently have:

- Reading ease and familiarity of words. All self-administered question-naires should be written at a sixth-grade reading level (many word processors have a feature that allows you to test the reading level). Interviewer-administered or telephone administered questions should not use large words and should use simple sentence structures. Also be very careful no to use terms or abbreviations that may not be familiar to the participants. For example:

Confusing question		Better question
	→	
	→	
	→	

- Order of questions. Sensitive questions should be placed at the end of the survey. This will increase the number of people who will answer them (you will have already established a bit of rapport by the time you get to those), and will prevent possible negative feelings caused by the questions to interfere with the way people answer the rest of the survey. Potentially sensitive questions that should be placed at the end include:

  - Demographics (age, race, education, etc).
  - Income (this one is particularly sensitive to most US populations. Consider leaving it out unless you really need it, and then place it as the last question).
  - Questions about past abuse
  - Sensitive health issues, such as miscarriages, sexually transmitted infections, eating disorders, etc.
  - Other personal questions that most people would not discuss in casual conversation.

  Good questions to start the survey off with include:

  - Self-rated health ('Overall, would you say your health is excellent, good, fair or poor?'). This is an easy question for most people, and is actually a remarkably good predictor of future health outcomes.
  - Participation in certain programs or activities ('Have you ever participated in...' or 'How many times have you been involved in...')

- Ability to answer question appropriately. Confusing wording of a question or the lack of all relevant answer choices often lead to frustration on the part of participants and poor data for the project. Consider the following:

Problem question		Why it's a problem

Which type of insurance do you have?
  1. Medicare
  2. Medicaid
	→	Person may have a different type of insurance than the two listed. Should either provide more options (private insurance, etc), or rephrase the question ('Mark yes or no for whether you have either of the following two types of insurance')

What best describes your current employment situation?
  1. Employed full time
  2. Employed part time
  3. Employed in temporary position
  4. Not employed
	→	How should a person working in a temporary part-time job answer? Make sure question options are mutually exclusive (only one can apply to any single person), or allow respondents to select more than one answer.

Are you satisfied with your current primary health care provider?	→	What if the respondent doesn't have a current health care provider? Be careful not to make assumptions.
Do you support the proposed Health Initiative bill being voted on next week by congress?	→	It's likely many participants may have no idea what the initiative is about. Never assume people are aware of all the same information—explain everything.
Do you think that smoking should be banned in all restaurants and bars?	→	What if the respondent thinks smoking should be banned in restaurants, but not bars?

- Variability of answers. It is usually of very little use to you to have everyone answer a survey question in exactly the same way. More often than not, it means there was a problem with the question or that the question really didn't need to be asked in the first place. Consider the following:

> Please rate the quality of our program services:
>   1. Perfect
>   2. Good
>   3. Useless

It's pretty likely that almost everyone will answer 'good', but that doesn't really give you the information you wanted. Changing the options to allow more variability (Excellent, Good, Fair, Poor, Useless) would make the question much more useful.

- Prioritize questions to ask on the survey. The longer your survey, the greater the demand on your staff members and the harder it will be to get people to participate. It's therefore important to prioritize your evaluation needs, and eliminate all but the absolutely essential questions for your survey. It is best to keep surveys to about 10–15 min.

5. Ethics and confidentiality

Informed consent must be administered regardless of the format of the survey.

6. Pilot test & revise

- After writing the end-of-session questionnaire, you should ask a few clients or participants to take the questionnaire in exactly the same way that you plan to do on a larger scale later. Ask the people who agree to pilot test if they'd be willing to give you their feedback afterwards. What did they think of the questions? Did anything confuse or bother them? What were they thinking about when they answered certain questions the way they did?
- Pilot testing is important to determine whether your questions are being interpreted the way you want them to. Without this critical feedback, you risk implementing a full data-collection plan only to find out at the end that important questions were misread and you didn't get the information you wanted.
- You will almost certainly find room for improvement in the questionnaire after the pilot test. Most questionnaires or surveys end up being revised eight-ten times before they are good enough to actually implement. Be open to feedback and suggestions from other staff members and the participants themselves. If you think your questionnaire is ready to go on the first or even second revision, you probably haven't put enough effort into the pilot testing.

7. Administer the survey

8. Entering & coding data

9. Tips for overcoming roadblocks

Ensure better response

End of Session Questionnaires & Pre/Post Tests

End of session questionnaires and pre/post tests are basically very short self-administered surveys. End of session questionnaires are generally given to gather information about what participants thought about an activity or intervention. Some of the following are examples of what information can be gained through end-of-session questionnaires:

- **Type of people who are participating in sessions**. What age, educational level, income level, etc. do people participating in your program usually have? (Helps you determine if you're reaching your target population, or what types of people are being missed)
- **Participant satisfaction.** What did people think of the session? Were they happy with it? Do they have suggestions for improvement? (This can help you improve the format of the sessions).
- **Participant evaluation of presenters.** How good did the presenter/educator/clinician/case worker do? Did the participant find the person knowledgeable, friendly, helpful? (this can help the presenter improve their skills for future sessions).
- **What participants think they gained from the session.** Note that you cannot find out what participants **actually** gained, only what they **think** they gained. Did they feel that they learned anything valuable?
- **Participants ideas/wants/needs for future sessions.** What did the participants want from the session that they didn't get? What would they like to see in future sessions? Do they have ideas for improvement? (Helps you plan future sessions).

Pre/post tests are generally given to measure a change in knowledge, attitudes, or beliefs after a participant engaged in a program activity. Note that you are measuring a *short-term* change with these. They can tell you the change that occurred during the activity or intervention, but not how much of that change will be retained in the future.

The steps to performing these methods are the same as for the self-administered survey. A few key things to note:

- Both types **must be kept extremely short.** Once you start stapling pages together, fewer people will be willing to take the time to go through it. Two-four pages is usually the most you want to have.
- The questions must be very simple and straight-forward. People will be answering the questions as they begin or finish an activity. It is unlikely that they will take much time to really think through the questions (or at least you can't expect that they will). If your questions are not extremely simple and easy to understand, it is likely that you won't get very good data.

Take some time to make the final questionnaire look pleasing. If you have a logo or a graphic, add it in. Make sure there is enough 'white space' (empty margins and spaces between questions). How the questionnaire looks is more important than you might think. Not only will a well-done questionnaire look more professional and make people take it more seriously, you want to make reading the questionnaire effortless!

- If it is not possible to survey all participants, you should try to implement a system of **random** selection of participants. This may mean every second or third group or client is asked to participate instead of every one, or one group per week rotating through the week (Monday's group this week, Tuesday's group next week, etc).
- Be careful to protect the privacy of participants. If the session was a group activity, make sure that your questionnaire does not contain any highly sensitive or personal information. Another option would be to provide a stamped envelope and allow people to take home the questionnaire and mail it back (though keep in mind you will get a much lower response rate through this method)
- Keep in mind that asking participants certain questions in a pre/post test design can actually influence what they pick up during the session. For example, asking about ways to prevent HIV before the session may make people more likely to pay attention to that part of an educational session than if they had not heard the question ahead of time.

Codebook Example

Variables	Definition of Indicators	Sources of data
Patient ID	Patient No: Number	Admitting Registration (Face sheet)
Age	Age: Number	Admitting Registration (Face sheet)
Sex	Male=0; Female=1	
Site	Residence site: Number (zip code)	Admitting Registration (Face sheet)
Race/ethnicity	Text (as recorded)	Admitting Registration (Face sheet)
Marital status	Single, divorced, widow, separated, married/in union	Admitting Registration (Face sheet)
Education	Last grade completed: 0–12	Clinical record: from 'Education'
Language	English, Spanish, Vietnamese, etc.	Clinical record: from 'Language'
Health insurance	0: self-paid; 1: charity care; 2:Medicaid; 3: Private insurance	Admitting Registration (Face sheet)

Health History	Diabetes: 0: No, 1:Yes	CVD record: from 'Medical history: #1: Diabetes'
	Hypertension: 0: No, 1:Yes	CVD record: from 'Medical history: #2: Hypertension'
	Heart Disease: Number: 0: No, 1:Yes	CVD record: from 'Medical history: #3: heart disease'
	Tobacco use:0: No, 1:Yes If yes, number of years use: Number	CVD record: from 'Medical history: #14: tobacco'
	Alcohol use: 0: No, 1:Yes If yes, number of years use: Number	CVD record: from 'Medical history: #15: alcohol'
Attitude	Desire/motivation to learn: 0: No, 1:Yes	Health education record: from 'Multidisciplinary patient/family education documentation sheet': 'Barrier to Learning'
	Immediate or strong interest: 0: No, 1:Yes	Health education record: from 'Health education needs and instruction checklist'

Appendix 2
Worksheets

Contents

Worksheet 1

Defining the Problem

What is the problem in the community that this program will address?

_____

_____

_____

How did you become aware of this issue?

_____

_____

_____

Who is directly affected?	How are they affected?

What are some possible reasons for this issue?	Why do these reasons exist?

How has this issue changed over the past several years? *(general trend in community)*	What influences have led to the changes?
(who is affected)	
(funding levels—public or private sources)	
(attention paid—media, schools, other)	
(similar changes elsewhere in country?)	
(Other)	

Who else is working on this?   What have they done?   Has it been successful?

Worksheet 2
Prioritizing Objectives & Indicators

GOAL of program:

Apply the 'SMART' test to each objective

Specific Does the objective mention details such as time, persons, and places?	**Measurable** Does the wording of the objective lead to an obvious way of measuring	**Attainable** Is the objective realistic given the time-frame and resources of the project?	**Related to goal:** Will achieving the objective directly assist in reaching the program	**Time-bound** Does the objective specify the time frame in which it is expected to be met?

Objective	Specific?	Measurable?	Attainable?	Related to goal?	Time-Bound?	Priority (Importance to goal) H-High M-Moderate L-Low — Priority of objective	Indicator(s) for objective	Data collection 0-Data already available 1-Easy to collect 2-Possible 3-Difficult — Ease of data collection	Priority of Indicator 1-Critical to objective 2-Important 3-Can do Without — Priority of indicator	Overall score (H,M, or L – and sum of previous two columns ex:. *M-1*) Overall priority score

Objective	S?	M?	A?	R?	T?	Priority of objective	Indicator(s) for objective	Easy of data collection	Priority of indicator	Overall priority score

Worksheet 3
Developing a Conceptual Framework

An empty conceptual framework looks like the figure below. It is easiest to start with the impact, then to fill in the background, mediating variables, program interventions, and then intermediate outcomes.

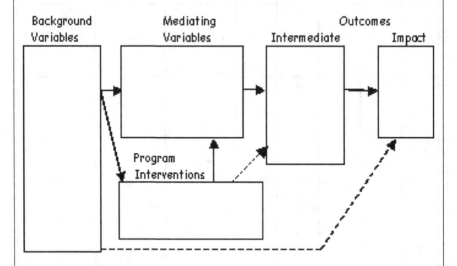

Step 1: Fill in the expected final impact of the program
The box for "impact" is basically a measure of your overall program goal. What are the things that your program hopes to change in the long term?

Phrase the expected impact in a neutral way that can be measured. For example, do not state "improved levels of vaccination among children." What if there was a *decline* in levels of vaccination rather than an improvement? It's not really the "improvement" you want to measure, it's just the rate of vaccination. The better way to phrase it would be, "vaccination rate among children."

Expected final impact(s):   *(Example: Systolic diastolic blood pressure among adults in program)*

Step 2: Fill in the important background variables
The easiest next step is to go back to the beginning and fill in the background variables. List all of the factors that can influence the final impact you listed above and can affect whether people access your services or not. Remember that background factors are aspects of your target population *before* they access your program services. Generally, they are not things that can be altered by your program.

Do *not* list attitudes, knowledge, beliefs or behaviors. All of these items can be altered, and will go in different boxes of the framework. Consider the following list of possible background factors. Check off those that are also relevant to your program. Be careful to list *only* those factors that are important in understanding how your program will influence change.

❑ Age	❑ Urban/rural residence	❑ Health/Medical history
❑ Sex/Gender	❑ Duration of residence in area	❑ History of healthcare access
❑ Race/ethnicity	❑ Duration of residence in USA	❑ Insurance status
❑ Primary language	❑ Domestic abuse	❑ Mental health/depression
❑ Education level	❑ History of physical abuse	❑ Smoking history/habits
❑ Marital status	❑ History of sexual abuse	❑ Pregnancy
❑ Income	❑ History of drug use	❑ Date of menarche
❑ Employment status	❑ Social support/networks	❑ Date of menopause
❑ Sexual orientation	❑ Transportation issues	❑ Number of children
❑ Height	❑ Living arrangements	❑ Number of pregnancies

❑ Other: _____ ❑ Other: _____
❑ Other: _____ ❑ Other: _____
❑ Other: _____ ❑ Other: _____
❑ Other: _____ ❑ Other: _____

Step 3: Fill in the mediating variables
Mediating variables are the knowledge, attitudes, and beliefs of your target population. Do *not* list behaviors here. Behaviors go in the intermediate outcomes box. This box is for all of the things that people know, think, or believe that *lead* them to do (or not do) certain behaviors.

Knowledge items (what people know or need to know):	(*Example: Aware of risk factors for CVD*)

Attitude items (what people feel or perceive)   (*Example: Perceived benefits of physical exercise*)

Belief items (what people believe or don't believe):   (*Example: Beliefs about food & family structure*)

Step 4: List the program interventions

Here, you simply list all of the activities that your program will perform, or service that it will provide, in order to affect the mediating variables and the outcomes.

Program activities or services: (*Example: CVD educational group sessions*)

Step 5: Decide on the expected intermediate outcomes
Write in what you expect to the short-term outcomes of your program. These are *behaviors* that you expect to see fairly soon after starting the program, and that could ultimately lead to the final impact from step 1.

Intermediate outcomes: *(Example: Increased physical exercise by at least 15 minutes per day))*

Step 6: Give your framework a descriptive title
Give a title to your conceptual framework that mentions your program and what the framework shows.

Title:

Step 7: Transfer the answers above to the conceptual framework diagram
An empty diagram is on the next page. Transfer only those variables you mentioned above that you believe are important to understanding how the program is intended to have an impact.

Step 8: Read through the framework
Read through the framework and make sure it makes sense.
- Does each background variable have the potential to affect the mediating variables, the final outcome, and/or access to your program?
- Would changes in the mediating variables lead to changes in the intermediate outcomes?
- Do the intermediate outcomes lead directly to the impact outcome?
- Are your program interventions able, at least in theory, to alter the mediating variables?

Note that it is possible for your program interventions to affect the intermediate outcomes (behaviors) directly – without first altering the mediating variables (knowledge and beliefs). This is not common, however, as usually behavior change only occurs after a change in knowledge, attitudes or beliefs have occurred. The dashed arrow from interventions to intermediate outcomes represents the small possibility of such an effect occurring.

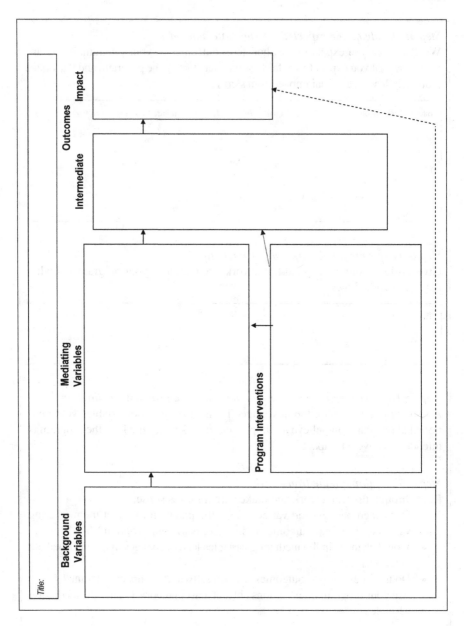

Worksheet 4
Informed Consent

Sample informed consent for a face-to-face activity (survey, focus group, interview, etc). Give a copy of the form to the participant, and keep the signed copy in your records.

Consent form for participation in evaluation

You are being asked to participate in an evaluation of the *[Program Name]* program. The evaluation is being conducted by *[Project Director or head evaluator]* in order to improve the *[name]* program. You were chosen to participate in this evaluation *[tell them why they were selected—random selection, because they use the services, etc]*. As a participant in this evaluation, you will be asked to *[tell them what tasks—fill out a survey, join in a group discussion, etc]*.

We will keep any information or answers you give us private at all times. Your information will be combined with information we receive from other people who participate in the evaluation. We will never use your name in any report or in connection with the information you give us. *[If asking people to join in a focus group, mention here how you cannot guarantee that other participants will keep the information private once they leave the discussion]*.

You do not have to participate in the evaluation. If you decide not to participate, it will not affect the services you receive from *[program name]* or your relationship with the organization in any way. If you agree to participate, you may change your mind at any time or refuse to answer any question.

If you have questions about the program or this evaluation, you can contact *[Project director, lead evaluator, or other contact person]* at *[phone number]*.

Your signature below states that you have read this form and understand it.

_____
Participant's signature   ❏ Agree to participate
                                                     ❏ Do not agree to participate

_____
Date

Sample informed consent for over-the-phone surveys

Hi. I'm *[name of caller]* calling from the *[Program name]*. We're calling *[fill in—clients, community members, residents of (town), etc]* to ask their opinions about *[fill in—our program, some health issues, etc]*. We'll use the answers we get to *[fill in purpose—evaluate our program and improve our services, etc]*

Your number was chosen randomly from a list of all residents/clients *[or fill in method of selection]*. Your participation is voluntary. Your answers will be combined with answers from other participants, and your name and information will be kept private. You can refuse to answer any question or stop the survey at any time. The survey will take about *[fill in estimated time of completion]* to complete. May we begin?

At the end of the survey:

[Name of program director, lead evaluator, or other contact] is in charge of this evaluation. Would you like *[name]*'s phone number or address in case you have questions about this survey or the evaluation?

Worksheet 5

Summary Table: Data Sources, Collection and Storage

	How	When	By Whom	In what form	Where	By Whom
Background i.e., Socio-demographic Health History	Example: Individual Clinic chart					
Mediating Psychosocial i.e., knowledge, attitudes	Example: Questionnaires					
Program Activities i.e., clinical test, education provided	Example: Program logs or records					
Intermediate outcomes Behavior i.e., adherence to health recommendations	Example: Questionnaires					
Final outcomes Physiological measures i.e., blood pressure	Example: Individual Clinic chart					

Index

Printed in the United States
By Bookmasters